WORKING-CLASS PATIENTS
AND THE
MEDICAL ESTABLISHMENT

TO
CATHERINE

Working-Class Patients and the Medical Establishment

Self-help in Britain
from the mid-nineteenth century to 1948

DAVID G. GREEN

Gower/Maurice Temple Smith

Published by
Gower Publishing Company Limited,
Gower House,
Croft Road,
Aldershot,
Hants GU11 3HR
England

Green, David
  Working-class patients and the medical
  establishment
  1. Social medicine—Great Britain
  2. Medical economics—Great Britain
  —History—19th century 3. Medical
  economics—Great Britain—History
  —20th century
  I. Title
  362.1'0941 RA418.3.G7

ISBN 0 85117 263 6

Typeset in 11 on 12 point Times by Tellgate Ltd, Swinton Street, London WC1
Printed and bound in Great Britain by Biddles Ltd, Guildford and King's Lynn

Contents

Tables

Abbreviations

AMC	Annual Moveable Conference
AOF	Ancient Order of Foresters
BMA	British Medical Association
BMJ	British Medical Journal
FSMA	Friendly Societies Medical Alliance
FSMI	Friendly Societies Medical Institute
GMC	General Medical Council
MOH	Ministry of Health
NCFS	National Conference of Friendly Societies
NDFS	National Deposit Friendly Society
PMSA	Provincial Medical and Surgical Association
PRO	Public Record Office
RFS	Chief Registrar of Friendly Societies
SWMA	South Wales and Monmouthshire Alliance of Medical Aid Societies

Preface

I am very grateful to the British Medical Association for granting me access to pre-war committee records. I am equally grateful to the Leicester Medical Society and to Dr K.F.C. Brown for making available library manuscripts. Thanks are also due to countless local librarians and museum curators for answering my letters about friendly society medical institutes.

I would also like to say a very big thank you to all those people who replied to my letters in the *Yorkshire Evening Press*, the *Eastern Daily Press*, and the *Luton News*. In particular I am grateful to Dr M.C. Barnet, and Mr E. Goodall for information about the York Friendly Societies Medical Institute; to the *Eastern Daily Press*, Mr M.W. Eagleton, Miss B.K. Rich, M.W.J. Tythcott, Mrs Allen (former dispenser to the Norwich FSMI), Mr H.R. Flack, Mrs B.M. Cross, Mrs N. Berry, Mrs E.W. Butcher, Mr W.J. Peck, and above all to Mr C.J. Waring (the former secretary of the Norwich FSMI) for information about the Norwich Friendly Societies Medical Institute. May I also thank Mrs E. Meakins, Mr A.E. Bodsworth, Ann M. Scales, Mrs E. Mead, Mrs E.M. Fairclough, Mr G.D.J. Lamb, and Mr J.G. Dony for information about the Luton Friendly Societies Medical Institute; and Mr L.H. Goldsmith for information about the Lowestoft Friendly Societies Medical Institute.

The friendly societies have offered every assistance in making available records and allocating time for interviews. May I particularly thank D.W. Nichols of the Hearts of Oak Benefit Society; Mr W.H. Robinson of the Grand United Order of Oddfellows; Mr Reg. Henry, the Grand Secretary of the Independent Order of Oddfellows, Manchester Unity; Alan V. Hall, secretary of Manchester Unity's Loyal John Barras Lodge in

Gateshead; R.W. Pollard, Mrs M.D. Newton, and Mr W.G. Cooper of the Ancient Order of Foresters; Mr R. Kirkland, Newcastle and North East Secretary of the Ancient Order of Foresters; and Peter Madders, the secretary of the National Conference of Friendly Societies.

Among colleagues I have received helpful criticisms from Norman Dennis, Professor Rudolf Klein, Sir Reginald Murley, Lord (Ralph) Harris of High Cross, Maurice Temple Smith, and above all from Arthur Seldon. It is impossible to thank Arthur Seldon enough for the support, encouragement and help he has provided over a period of several months. Needless to say, the responsibility for any remaining errors or omissions is mine alone.

Financially the study has been supported partly by the Nuffield Foundation and partly by the Institute of Economic Affairs. Without this financial support, particularly from the IEA, it would not have been possible to complete the study.

Finally, I am very grateful to Elaine Scotland, who typed the early drafts of the book, and above all to my wife, Catherine, who typed the final version, and helped with the dreadful chore of proof-reading.

November 1984

1
Introduction

Victorian Britain tends to be thought of as the heyday of *laissez-faire*. In this view, welfare was the province of a restrictive Poor Law and burgeoning private charity; and the production of goods and services the province of profit-seeking commercial companies. But the Victorian age was not only the heyday of 'bourgeois' values. Existing alongside was a clear working-class alternative, aiming to replace the hated Poor Law and the largesse of the well-to-do with the mutual aid of the friendly society and the trade union branch. Through the trade unions workers would win the wages necessary to sustain a decent existence, and through the friendly societies they would organize their own welfare services – social insurance, medical care, even housing loans. The profit motive, too, was to be supplanted: in the factory by the mutuality of the workers' co-op; and in retailing by the co-op store.

Not all these working-class hopes were realized, but the friendly societies, the trade unions and the co-op stores were successful and offered a fraternal alternative to the sometimes cold world of commercial calculation. Particularly striking is the success of the friendly societies, whose social insurance and primary medical care schemes had attracted at least three-quarters of manual workers well before the end of the nineteenth century. Until the 1911 National Insurance Act every neighbourhood of every town was dotted with friendly society branches, each with their own doctor, who had usually been elected by a vote of all the members assembled in the branch meeting. In most large towns the friendly societies had also established medical institutes combining doctors' living accommodation, surgery and a dispensary. These embryo health centres employed full-time salaried medical practitioners, full-time dispensers, and nursing staff under the management of a committee elected by all members.

The friendly societies were so successful that their arrangements for social insurance and primary medical care formed the model for the early welfare state. But this, ironically, was their undoing. The 1911 National Insurance Act was originally seen by Lloyd George, who charted it through Parliament, as a way of extending the benefits of friendly society membership, already freely chosen by the vast majority of workers, to *all* citizens, and particularly to those so poor they could not afford the modest weekly contributions. But on its way through the House of Commons the original Bill was radically transformed by powerful vested interests hostile to working-class mutual aid. The organized medical profession had long resented the dominance of the medical consumer, and particularly resented working-class control of medical 'gentlemen'. The BMA were equally anxious to obtain more pay and, above all, higher status for doctors. Working-class fraternalism also had another arch-enemy: the commercial insurance companies. They had long disliked the competition of the non-profit friendly societies and saw the 1911 National Insurance Bill as a threat to their business. They were organized in a powerful trade association, called the 'Combine'. The BMA and the Combine formed a temporary alliance to extract concessions from the government at the expense of the friendly societies. The essence of working-class social insurance was democratic self-organization: amendments to the Bill obtained by the BMA and the Combine undermined it. Doctors' pay had been kept within limits that ordinary manual workers could afford: under pressure, the government doubled doctors' incomes and financed this transfer of wealth from insured workers to the medical profession by means of a regressive poll tax, flat-rate National Insurance contributions.

The unhappy outcome of legislation initially intended to extend to all citizens the benefits of friendly society membership, already freely chosen by the vast majority, was a victory for the political muscle of the Combine and the BMA. They achieved a very considerable transfer of wealth and power from the relatively poor working class to the professional class.

Working-class Mutual Aid and 'Market Failure'

The research for this book was originally undertaken in order to write a history of working-class self-organized medical care. But as the investigation progressed it became obvious that the findings contradicted certain prevailing theories. The dominant academic view is that attempts by ordinary people to obtain health care for themselves, without the help of the state, are bound to suffer from a number of serious 'market failures':

1. *Monopoly:* The market for health is particularly vulnerable to monopoly – the medical profession can organize against the consumer to raise prices and to minimize accountability for medical wrongdoing.

2. *Consumer ignorance:* Because of his superior knowledge, the doctor always faces the consumer as the dominant party, a problem made worse by medical advance. Some economists contend that this knowledge imbalance gives rise to an 'agency relationship': the doctor is in reality both the demander, advising the patient how much to consume, and the supplier. For this reason normal freedom of choice cannot be exercised. Usually scholars who take this view also regard the market as inherently vulnerable to monopoly. But there is also a second group, chiefly sociologists, who are aware that free markets have sometimes produced *consumer* dominance. Their criticism is that historically dominance by ill-informed consumers meant low standards of health care, a problem which had to be remedied by the government intervention of 1911.

3. *Neglect of the poor and chronic sick:* If the market does not neglect the poor and chronic sick altogether, they receive an inferior service.

4. *Externalities:* There are negative externalities or third-party effects requiring government regulation, notably that the doctor and the patient may ignore the exposure of others to contagious disease.

5. *Lack of provision of public goods:* Some health care is a 'public good' which must be supplied by government, notably the elimination of contagious disease.

6. *The perverse incentives of insurance:* Demand for health care is more uncertain than for most other products and in practice this has meant that insurance has played a major role in

health care funding. But there are special difficulties about health insurance: (a) once insured the individual has a reduced incentive to avoid health care costs, and more importantly, once premiums have been paid the individual has an incentive to initiate the delivery of health care, that is to 'get his money's worth'; and (b) where a third party controls payment, neither the doctor nor the patient may have an incentive to contain costs.

The friendly societies did not seem to fit this theory. Manual workers, often with little to call their own, had evolved by their united endeavours organizations for the supply of primary medical care that were not surpassed anywhere in the world. Their successful pioneering efforts were only undermined when the government of the day fell under the power of a political alliance of big business and the organized medical profession.

In studying how this came about this book will focus on the primary medical care market in Britain in two main periods: (a) before the 1911 National Insurance Act, when there was a free market for all but the beneficiaries of the Poor Law; and (b) from 1913 to 1948, when there was a state medical benefit scheme for those (largely men) insured under the 1911 Act alongside free-market provision for the non-insured – the wives, the children, and some of the elderly.

The New Left

For much of this century, and certainly since the Second World War, almost all shades of political opinion accepted that the state should be the chief instrument of social reform. During the 1970s some Left-wing intellectuals began to question whether the state should play such a prominent part in socialist thought. Was there not, some of them asked, a tradition of 'decentralized socialism'? They had in mind the fraternal organizations evolved by manual workers in the nineteenth century: the friendly societies, trade unions, and co-ops. Socialists in Britain began to discuss the merits of the market more openly, and hard on the heels of 'market socialism' – long discussed in the Eastern bloc – came the 'social market' of the SDP.

Yet a great many people who identified with the Left felt uneasy about this. Some who found themselves rationally convinced by the arguments felt a sense of guilt, even shame, about their change of mind. Suppose the worst fears of the traditional Left were realized? What would happen to the poor? What would happen to housing policy, education, health and social security? People might die in the streets and doctors demand cash in advance as patients lay bleeding; ruthless landlords might evict at will, and the children of the poor remain illiterate and innumerate, while the poor themselves fell below subsistence level.

Fears such as these are still very much to the fore, and those who advocate the market-socialist solution have yet to respond satisfactorily. This book does not examine directly all the evidence that needs to be taken into account in calculating the probable effects of a programme of reform of our medical services. It does not investigate health care in other countries in which the state already plays a smaller role, and it does not examine the private sector in Britain today. Nor does it investigate the hospital sector in Britain before the NHS. These are areas which other scholars have studied. This book focuses instead on the most neglected part of the evidence: how the great majority of the population, manual workers and their families, fared in the system that existed for a hundred years and more before the NHS. What actually happened when, at one particular time in history, working-class patients set out to organize health care for themselves?

2
Professional Monopoly Power

This book tests two theories which attempt to explain how professional monopoly power arises. The first is the 'market vulnerability' theory that a free market in health care *as such* is inherently prone to monopoly. Professor Alan Maynard, for instance, contends that the 'natural inclination of a competitive market is for it to become monopolistic' (1982, p. 495). And for Professor A.J. Culyer, markets are 'always and everywhere so imperfect that the marketeers' image of the market for health is a completely irrelevant description of an unattainable Utopia' (1982, p. 27). Among the leading imperfections he identifies is the tendency to monopoly: 'It seems that a strongly organized professional monopoly that controls entry to the profession, terms of service, permitted forms of advertising, disciplinary procedure, etc., is a *universal* characteristic of all developed countries (wherever they lie on the liberal–collective spectrum)' (emphasis in original; 1982, p. 37).

Generally academics who take this view believe that to protect consumers the power of the state should be used as a countervailing power. It should at least regulate the private monopoly and better still take over the service and run it as a government monopoly. Professor Culyer, for instance, argues that because of the tendency of the health care market to monopoly there is 'at least a *prima facie* case for introducing a countervailing bargaining power, in the form of the state, in the determination of wages and salaries' (1982, p. 37).

The second of the explanatory theories I will test is the contrary view that it is not the free market in itself which necessarily gives rise to monopoly power, but rather the ease with which producers can use the power of the state to enforce their monopoly. I will call this the 'state capture' theory. D.S. Lees, for example, argues that monopoly gains will be 'potentially largest where a profession has achieved legal or effective monopoly through the political process' (1966, p. 46). Proponents of this view generally contend that it is the duty of government not to allow the state to be used to create new monopolies or reinforce existing ones. Libertarian writers further argue that monopolies cannot exist for long in a free market (see e.g. Friedman, D., 1978, p. 60; see also Hayek, 1960, p. 266). But if they are enforced by government they are more difficult to displace. In this view, there are two main ways in which private organizations of producers use the state. The first is to seek to establish official government regulatory agencies to control prices when their cartels have failed. The second is to extract concessions from interventionist governments which are seeking their cooperation. Producers may encourage or plan such intervention, or their actions may be simply opportunistic.

The theories will be tested throughout the life of the modern medical profession. No definite date can be given, but it is unrealistic to think of the various persons who specialized in health care as resembling today's medical profession until the 1830s at the earliest. I will, therefore, begin this investigation in the 1830s. In the remainder of this chapter I will examine medical care delivery in the market, excluding, that is, Poor Law medical care. In Chapter 3 I will survey the early efforts made to abuse the power of the state.

Was there a professional monopoly in the medical marketplace which existed prior to the 1911 National Insurance Act? Medical care was being provided in a variety of ways at the turn of the century. Apart from the Poor Law, they fall into three main categories. First, a large section of the population obtained care free of charge through charities. Particularly in London and the larger towns, they used the outpatient departments of the voluntary hospitals; and some used the free dispensaries where these existed. Second, many sought medical care as private patients and paid a fee to the doctor of their choice. The fees charged varied according to income, with rent taken as the chief test of income (see below p. 90). In the third category were the wide variety of insurance schemes, commonly called contract practice. Treatment under these schemes was usually based on the payment of a fixed annual capitation fee. The various types of scheme are identified in a report of the medico-political committee of the BMA, published in 1905.

I propose to proceed by searching from the 1830s until the 1911 Act for evidence of professional monopoly control of primary medical care. I will focus on the conflict which emerged between organized medical consumers and the organized profession. Plainly, if the profession failed to get its way against consumer organizations, any theory asserting the inherent and inevitable tendency of medical markets to professional monopoly stands refuted, and some alternative theory has to be found.

Types of Contract Practice

Each type of contract practice was based on the principle of the flat-rate annual contribution, usually payable quarterly but sometimes weekly or fortnightly, entitling the contributor to any number of consultations during the period covered. Some such clubs were based at factories, others were organized by charities; some were run on commercial lines, some by individual doctors, some by local associations of doctors, and some by the friendly societies. By far the most important numerically were the friendly society schemes.

Works Clubs (Medical Aid Societies)

A number of doctors were employed by works clubs. Workers at a factory or mine arranged with their employer to deduct an agreed sum from their pay for the provision of medical attendance and medicines for themselves, and usually for their families. Some doctors were paid a fixed salary, others an annual amount per patient. In some cases the employer himself engaged a medical practitioner to attend his workers, but by the turn of the century it was more usual for the selection of a doctor to be left to the workers themselves. The general body of employees at a factory or mine, or working in a particular district, chose their medical attendant in a general meeting. Frequently committees were appointed by the workers to manage the club.

Some hospitals were run on works-club lines. An infirmary in North Staffordshire was supported by penny-a-week contributions deducted from the pay packets of workers at the local factories and iron works. The hospital doctors were unpaid and objected to local workers coming to the hospital as outpatients for free attention. Many, it was said, were paid £1 to £3 a week, and it was felt they could afford fees (*BMJ*, 17 August 1867, p. 139). Often in such cases the hospital outpatients department functioned as a club for the whole family, as in Swansea (*Lancet*, 28 December 1895, p. 1671). The most resilient of the works clubs were the 'medical aid societies' founded by the miners and steelworkers of the Welsh valleys.

Provident Dispensaries
The provident dispensaries were semi-charities, funded partly by the contributions of beneficiaries and partly by the charitable donations of the (non-benefiting) honorary members. Provident or self-supporting dispensaries developed out of the free dispensaries, many of which had been established during the course of the eighteenth century. Free dispensaries were felt to create a permanently dependent section of the population. Provident dispensaries, therefore, aimed to enable the poor to make as much of a contribution as they could to the cost of their medical care, with the balance to be supplied by charity. A movement for self-supporting dispensaries developed in the 1820s under the encouragement of H.L. Smith, a surgeon who founded the Southam Dispensary in Warwickshire in 1823. His intention was to replace both the free dispensaries and club practice. The original plan was for all the surgeons in a district to join the scheme, with patients having the right of choice between them. The whole family was to be covered, and doctors were to be paid by the case and not by capitation fee. Medicines were to be supplied, not by the doctors, but by dispensers employed by the provident dispensary.

Three classes of member were distinguished. Class one, or free members, were those who were willing and able to be self-dependent as long as they pooled their resources, but who as individual families could not have afforded to pay a doctor's fees. Class two members were those who were willing but unable to be self-reliant. They required the assistance of the honorary members, who paid half a guinea a year for each patient they wished to support. The third class of members were the paupers, who were admitted not by their own free decision, nor by the recommendation of an honorary member, but by contract with the parish overseer. By 1829 the movement had led to the establishment of at least six dispensaries in the Midlands, including one at Birmingham (Smith, 1819; 1830; Second Annual Report of the Southam Dispensary, 1825). By the 1850s few paupers were being provided for by provident dispensaries, most of the members were free subscribers or charity patients. By this time the most successful dispensaries were at Derby and Coventry (Rumsey, 1856, pp. 159–62). In 1906 the Coventry Provident **Dispensary still had over 20,000** members (RCPL, 1909, Appendix XIV).

Like most of the other provident dispensaries the income of the Northampton Provident Dispensary was derived from three sources: donations, subscriptions (by honorary members who did not use the services), and the contributions of 'free members'. The free members paid 1d a week if they were over fourteen and ½d if they were younger, but a man, wife and children could be covered for 2d per week. There were four surgeons, who would visit homes where necessary. Medicines were provided by the dispensary (*Lancet*, 1850, pp. 89–90). By the 1860s doctors' conditions compared favourably with those obtaining in some other towns. The Northampton dispensary had an income limit to exclude the well-off and paid its three surgeons £1,027 a year for attending 3,807 members. Conditions at Birmingham were less favourable. The Cannon Street Male Provident Institution paid its nine surgeons a total of £836 for attending 6,638 members. The Birmingham doctors were required to supply drugs and appliances, whilst the Northampton doctors were not (*BMJ*, 13 July 1867, p. 28; 28 December 1867, p. 594).

By 1905 the BMA was complaining that advantage had been taken of provident dispensaries by persons who were 'quite able to pay for medical attendance' (BMA, CPR, 1905, p. 20). They objected to the fact that the dispensaries were managed by lay committees appointed by the honorary members, and that the pay was too low. The arrangement of the Sunderland Provident Dispensary was reasonably typical. After payment of an admission fee, each adult paid 4d per month; a man and a wife, 8d; and a man, wife plus children under sixteen, 1s. These fees included payment for medicines prescribed by institute doctors. Medical officers were paid a percentage of the total income after expenses had been met. Three fifths of the income went direct to the medical officers, plus two thirds of any surplus remaining after the payment of expenses (*BMJ*, 23 March 1895, p. 657).

Medical Aid Companies

Some contract medical practice was organized on commercial lines. Medical aid companies were promoted by non-medical persons, as a commercial speculation for the direct or indirect profit of the promoters. Such companies differed from the friendly societies and works clubs, which were promoted for the benefit of members and their dependants, and the promoters had little in common with the honorary members of provident dispensaries, who themselves contributed to a charity for the assistance of the poor. One example of these commercial companies was the National Medical Aid Company, which offered medical attendance as an inducement to obtain life assurance business (*Lancet*, 5 October 1895, p. 875).

Doctors' Clubs

There were also a large number of clubs organized by the doctors themselves. Many employed collectors to recruit new members as well as to call regularly for patients' contributions. This made the arrangement 'open to objection, particularly when the collector was paid by commission on the amount collected'. Many medical practitioners criticized the doctors' clubs. One described the 'penny a week club' as 'the curse of the medical profession'. The collector's commission was occasionally as low as 5 per cent but sometimes reached 25 per cent, and in one instance a collector received 25 per cent of the weekly payments, together with the whole of the first week's subscription.

The BMA's survey of members revealed that many doctors were sympathetic to such clubs:

The family club run by the doctor himself is a necessity. He can be dismissed at a moment's notice very often from a Friendly Society. The individual member of his own club, if he has a complaint to make, does it personally. The doctor is free from the supervision, and, as I have found, the impertinence of the committee of the Friendly Society. The patients in a family club look up to him personally. In the Friendly Society club he is very often treated as a servant. The smallest infringement of their rules means a complaint and a visit from the committee. The doctor of a family club can make his own terms. . .

In my opinion the most satisfactory form of contract practice is the private club: one can accept those who really cannot pay full fees, and can refuse those who can afford to pay properly, and there is no committee to trouble one (BMA, CPR, pp. 21–2).

Public Medical Services
Public medical services were rather like provident dispensaries. The chief difference was that provident dispensaries were controlled by lay committees, whereas public medical services were 'under the entire control of the medical profession'. In 1905 public medical services were a recent phenomenon. Usually they had been founded by the local branch of the BMA to combat provident dispensaries, medical aid societies, or friendly societies (BMA, CPR, p. 23).

The Friendly Society Schemes
The friendly societies were self-governing, fraternal associations for mutual aid. Each family paid into a common fund which was used to provide sick pay in the event of illness or accident and a benefit to the survivor at death. The societies also supplied medical care and made available practical or financial help for members facing temporary distress. Most societies also provided convalescent homes, usually by several lodges pooling their resources. London friendly societies had their own convalescent home, as did those in the Midlands and the North East, whose members paid 1s 0d a year towards the Grange-over-Sands home (*Lancet*, 17 September 1887, p. 599; *Oddfellows Magazine*, 22 September 1889, p. 524; June 1895, pp. 187–8).

There were several different types of friendly society, but here I will identify only four. The simplest type was the local dividing society (sometimes called a slate club or tontine). Once a year, usually just before Christmas, any surplus remaining in the fund was divided among the members. Secondly, there were the large federations or affiliated orders, such as Manchester Unity and the Ancient Order of Foresters. These comprised autonomous local branches united under a common set of rules. At the turn of the century they were by far the most popular form of friendly society. Thirdly, there were deposit societies.

They were national organizations with no branches, which combined saving with social insurance. Each claim for benefit was met, not solely by a payment from the society's accumulating sick fund, but partly from the common fund and partly from the member's personal interest-earning savings account (usually in the ratio 2 to 1). Finally, there were centralized societies without branches, like the Hearts of Oak Benefit Society, which paid sick pay from an accumulating fund.

Among the great variety of arrangements made for the supply of medical care three proved most popular: the lodge system, medical institutes, and approved panels.

Lodge practice: The traditional system in the large federations was for each branch to employ a single medical officer. Usually the appointment was made by a free vote of all the members present at a general meeting. Sometimes doctors were invited to submit tenders before the election. In some areas several medical officers were appointed to a branch or a combination of branches, and the members then enjoyed a free choice among the available doctors. Sometimes medical officers were appointed at the pleasure of the branch, and sometimes for a fixed period of three months, six months, or a year.

The medical officer's duties were threefold. First, he would examine candidates for lodge membership. Second, he would examine members who were sick to determine whether or not they should receive sick pay. Third, he would provide medical attendance and medicines for each lodge member in return for a fixed annual capitation fee, usually payable quarterly.

Medical institutes: Lodge doctors were usually only part time and in some localities friendly society members felt they neglected contract patients in favour of private patients. Moreover, wives and children were not generally covered by lodge practice. From about 1869 a movement developed to overcome these problems by founding medical institutes to employ full-time medical officers serving the whole family. Groups of lodges spontaneously banded together, raised funds and purchased or rented premises. Organization was under the control of a committee of delegates which appointed one or more full-time medical officers, who usually received a fixed salary plus free accommodation. Medical officers' duties usually included general medical and surgical attendance, but not the dispensing of medicines. Dispensing was carried out by the medical institute's own dispenser to ensure use of the highest quality drugs.

Approved panels: By the turn of the century the closed panel system was growing in popularity. Friendly society members appointed doctors to a panel from which members could choose their family doctor. To be eligible to join the panel, doctors were required to conform with the conditions laid down by the friendly society and particularly to accept prescribed fees. The most sophisticated scheme was that of the National Deposit Friendly Society.

Early Professional Action

The Provincial Medical and Surgical Association, founded in 1832, became the British Medical Association in 1855. The first organization to bear the name 'British Medical Association' was a rival body to the PMSA. The original BMA became defunct within a few years of its foundation, but in the 1830s it was a major rival to the PMSA.

One of the earliest targets of the organized medical profession was the Poor Law. After its reform in 1834 the general feeling among Poor Law administrators was that the Poor Law, including its medical service, had been wastefully administered. This led to considerable tightening up of the system, to which doctors took exception. Their campaign was led by the original British Medical Association, which had two main objections to the new Poor Law.

The first was the introduction of tendering for Poor Law medical posts. The second was the Poor Law commissioners' plan to establish independent medical clubs for non-paupers. Mechanics, artisans, domestic servants, and independent labourers were to be encouraged to join independent medical clubs. A scale of annual capitation fees was proposed in the Poor Law Report of 1836: 3s per single person; 4s per man and wife; 6d per child under sixteen. These plans were implemented in some areas amidst professional protests. Had these plans succeeded, the BMA believed, it would have 'entirely blasted the prospects of the humbler practitioner' (*Lancet*, 25 August 1838, pp. 751–63). In some localities guardians continued to encourage the development of clubs; and in others the BMA persuaded them to desist.

One of the earliest professional objections to independent medical clubs appeared in April 1837. In a leading article the *Lancet* opposed a semi-charitable 'penny club' in the Cricklade and Wootton Bassett Poor Law union (15 April 1837, p. 133). And in July the *Lancet* attacked the penny clubs and self-supporting dispensaries then being promoted by Mr H.L. Smith of Southam (15 July 1837, pp. 593–6).

These were objections to the semi-charitable clubs managed on behalf of the poor by the well-to-do, and usually by clergymen. Some doctors also objected to the self-managed friendly society schemes. In 1839, for instance, the Leeds Oddfellows were in dispute with their lodge surgeons, who felt that 2s 6d per year was too low. The Oddfellows responded to the doctors' demands by advertising in London for replacements (SCMPR, 1844, Q. 9078). Sometimes doctors tried to boycott contract practice altogether. In 1844 in Sunderland there were about sixty clubs with 4,500 members, some paying 2s a year, others 3s. In a pattern which was often to be repeated, thirty-five local GPs joined together to try to ban contract practice. They only needed two or three more colleagues to make the ban effective (SCMPR, 1844, Q. 9078). But they failed.

In the 1840s and 1850s the organized medical profession was not opposed to clubs as such, but doctors did seek 'considerable and immediate reform'. There were two main objections: the low pay, and the admission of members who could afford to pay higher fees. Doctors who were influential in the clubs were also urged as part of their 'humanizing mission' to discourage their poorer brethren from holding meetings in public houses (*Lancet*, 1849, p. 570; *Association Medical Journal*, 2 September 1853, p. 766; 7 October 1853, p. 888).

Doctors sought to exclude the wealthy by imposing an income limit on the clubs. Some clubs did include an income limit in their rules (e.g. *Lancet*, 1851, p. 359) but most did not. In 1845 one correspondent to the *Lancet* complained that 'well-nigh every general practitioner is either immediately or indirectly affected' by medical clubs. In the Pickering district of Yorkshire, tradesmen, innkeepers and farmers, who could well afford ordinary fees, were members. In June 1844 some doctors in the locality had formed the Medical Protection Association. Each member signed a pledge not to participate in contract practice. The local clubs retaliated by advertising for an outside doctor. Their original choice turned out to be unqualified, but he was quickly replaced by a qualified practitioner. Twelve months after the foundation of the MPA, unity among doctors had collapsed (*Lancet*, 1845, pp. 163–6).

Efforts to impose wage limits continued elsewhere. Doctors in the south-east branch of the BMA met in 1852 to try to impose a wage limit on the local clubs. Doctors signed a pledge not to work for clubs which failed to enforce a wage limit which would exclude workers earning in excess of 20s a week. There were four clubs in Canterbury. Three had modified their rules and the fourth club's decision was awaited. If it refused to comply, the medical officer planned to resign and no other local doctor would take his place. The outcome is unknown, but the doctors had enjoyed some success in coercing the other three clubs. One had been a branch of Manchester Unity, which, very unusually for Manchester Unity, had after 'some difficulty' agreed to change its by-laws. Fees do not seem to have been at issue. The annual fee was 4s 4d, a penny a week (*Association Medical Journal*, 22 July 1853, pp. 652–3).

The chief complaint of the doctors was that they were underpaid. In the 1840s competition was often vigorous and blamed on the overcrowded state of the profession. In Cheltenham in 1848, for instance, one doctor undercut another by nearly 30 per cent, offering to serve a club for 2s 6d per head per year instead of 3s 6d (*Lancet*, 1849, p. 102). The BMA put the blame for competition, not on the younger doctor starting out, but on the well-established and wealthy practitioner with a good income who took on assistants to do the club work for a comparative pittance (*Association Medical Journal*, 23 February 1853, pp. 825–6).

In the 1850s strong competition continued between members of the Society of Apothecaries, the Royal College of Surgeons, and the graduates of the medical schools. Complaints were voiced that new medical schools were being opened when the profession was already too full (*Lancet*, 27 March 1858, p. 332; *BMJ*, 8 February 1868, p. 135). The number of medical practitioners continued to expand throughout the century, and against this background it proved difficult to maintain effective professional combinations. Doctors' attempts to raise fees often met with total defeat.

At Alfreton in Derbyshire, for example, doctors banded together in 1856 to try to impose new conditions on local clubs: notably a minimum fee of 3s a year, and extra fees for accidents. A delegate meeting of thirty societies was called to discuss the new rules proposed by the doctors. They were rejected 'in toto', and advertisements were placed for different doctors (*Lancet*, 21 June 1856, p. 674; 30 August 1856, p. 226; 13 September 1856, pp. 314–5). Competition meant that in Wolverhampton in 1856 some medical men of many years experience were working for as little as 1s 0d per patient per year (*Lancet*, 4 October 1856, p. 396). And in Guisborough in Yorkshire a year later, fees were also 1s 0d (AOF, Court Old Abbey 603, *Laws*, 1857, rule VI). In the early 1850s the average weekly wage in wage-earning families was about 20s (Wood, 1962). Capitation fees varied a great deal from place to place, but according to the BMA the average was about 3s to 4s a year (*Association Medical Journal*, 23 September 1853, p. 825).

Professional Organization Grows

A more concerted effort at combination on a large scale took place in Birmingham in the late 1860s. In 1867 the annual meeting of the Birmingham and Midlands Counties branch of the BMA passed a resolution that club payments were too low. The movement for an increase was led by Dr Heslop. During his speech to the annual meeting he said he anticipated that: 'We shall obtain all that we have a fair claim to by argument, by conference with the authorities of the societies, and by discussion in the press, in the presence of a well-informed public.' He also called for a united effort on the part of the profession (*BMJ*, 22 June 1867, vol. 1, p. 745; 20 July 1867, p. 45; *Lancet*, 3 August 1867, p. 149). The campaign was supported by the *BMJ*, which complained that private medical fees had risen about 50 per cent since the 1830s, whilst annual club payments had remained stationary at 3s or even fallen to 2s 6d (6 July 1867, p. 8).

In December 1867 the Birmingham branch listed their grievances: (1) The great disproportion between the amount of work and pay. In addition to being available at surgeries, doctors were expected to make home visits, supply medicines and carry out operations. (2) Many club members could afford ordinary fees. Wealthy club members fell into two groups:

those who had begun poor and risen in life; and those who joined the clubs when already wealthy. This last group were strongly resented. (3) The requirement that doctors supply sick certificates to members often brought them into conflict with both members and club committees.

The doctors demanded the imposition of an income limit; a pay rise, with the minimum fee fixed at 5s per annum; and the levying of an additional fee for carrying out medical examinations prior to club entry (*BMJ*, 28 December 1867, pp. 594–5).

Initially the Birmingham doctors campaigned for a 5s minimum for every new appointment, but from March 1868 they pressed for all existing medical officers to be paid 5s. The doctors secured the support of the Birmingham newspapers. The *Birmingham Daily Gazette* called upon the friendly societies not to insist that market forces alone determine fees. Certainly doctors could be found in abundance to fill available places at well below 5s, but justice demanded that the doctors be better paid. Their expenses had risen considerably, whilst the ability of working men to pay more had also increased (*BMJ*, 11 January 1868, p. 38).

The response of the clubs was mixed. Some friendly societies considered establishing a new dispensary to employ a full-time doctor and undermine the doctors' campaign. Some accepted the 5s rate willingly, and many offered increases to 3s 6d or 4s. Many friendly society members felt that the doctors request for an increase was essentially 'fair' and called for a 'fair' response (*Lancet*, 24 October 1868, p. 549; *BMJ*, 1 February 1868, p. 104; *BMJ*, 10 October 1868, p. 407).

The Cannon Street Male Provident Institution, a provident dispensary, became notorious for its opposition to the doctors. At its annual meeting in January 1868 the doctors request for an increase was rejected, chiefly because eight doctors had offered to serve the club at 2s 6d. But the following month, under pressure from the BMA committee, six of the eight resigned (*BMJ*, 8 February 1868, p. 128). As a result, the club committee agreed to further discussion of the claim, and the doctors agreed to carry out their duties whilst discussions took place. This was applauded by the *BMJ* which felt sure that the local BMA committee would not approve of a strike which sought by 'intimidation and sudden inconvenience to force a decision' (*BMJ*, 15 February 1868, p. 152). A compromise was reached.

The Birmingham committee organized a pledge of solidarity and by February 1868 it had been signed by 168 doctors, with only a minority of Birmingham doctors declining (*BMJ*, 22 February 1868, p. 184). In Wolverhampton a similar declaration was signed by all but two doctors (*BMJ*, 14 March 1868, p. 253). In his annual address in 1868 the president reviewed progress since the previous annual meeting. As a mark of success he pointed out that two doctors had increased their annual earnings by £400. But he criticized the apathy of many doctors. Too many had been content 'to look on' while others fought. And too many had allowed themselves to be 'talked over by the claptrap nonsense of bad times', or 'the poor club members can't afford it' (*BMJ*, 11 July 1868, p. 34). During these years many other doctors wrote to the *BMJ* complaining about the lack of unanimity among colleagues (see e.g. *BMJ*, 17 August 1867, pp. 139–40; 31 August 1867, p. 196).

The move of the Birmingham doctors was soon being emulated all over the country. In May 1868 doctors at Southampton combined to raise fees (*BMJ*, 6 June 1868, p. 564; see also 25 April 1868, p. 409). Doctors at Oldbury in South Staffordshire also combined, but they met with a vigorous reaction. The clubs refused to budge and brought in three new doctors. In July the Oldbury doctors retaliated by ostracizing the newcomers: 'We pledge ourselves neither to meet them professionally nor socially; and we further pledge ourselves not to consent to meet in consultation any physician or surgeon who recognizes them' (*BMJ*, 11 July 1868, p. 32). Doctors in North Staffordshire had already begun a campaign to impose conditions on the clubs. The wealthy were to be excluded and a minimum fee imposed (*Lancet*, 2 February 1867, pp. 155–6). In 1869 the Shropshire Ethical Branch campaigned for a minimum fee of 5s, except for agricultural labourers earning 12s a week or less, who would pay 4s. About a hundred doctors pledged not to accept future appointments except on these terms (*BMJ*, 30 October 1869, p. 477).

By 1869 the *Lancet* was referring to the 'battle of the clubs', declaring it to be 'undecided' (*Lancet*, 1869, vol. 1, p. 60). But there was little or no hostility to contract practice as a principle. Sick club medical officers in Liverpool for example met in 1869 and expressed in resolutions their approval of sick benefit societies, and their desire to cooperate with 'provident mechanics and labourers' in procuring relief by such means. They also agreed that 4s should be the minimum rate, and that the well-to-do should be excluded altogether (*BMJ*, 14 August 1869, p. 187).

Also during 1869 doctors in the West Bromwich area applied to thirty-four societies for an increase in the prevailing 3s rate. In a response which was probably fairly typical, eighteen of these societies increased fees to 4s; seven to 5s; and in one case a new club was formed and paid 10s. Nine clubs refused to respond at all. One club initially increased its rate to 4s, but a little later, in June 1871, two doctors offered themselves at 3s and were appointed at the lower fee. Generally doctors felt that their agitation had been successful (*BMJ*, 10 June 1871, p. 626; 24 June 1871, p. 676).

The campaigns of the late 1860s and the 1870s were not characterized by the bitterness typical of later years. The *Lancet* found that many increases to 5s a year and more had been awarded 'without any undignified pressure, but from reasonable and courteous representations' (3 November 1877, p. 654). A doctor in Staffordshire, for instance, told the *Lancet* that on informing his own clubs that a number of Birmingham clubs were paying 5s, he had met with a good response. All had agreed to pay him 5s. He had served them for twenty-three years and initially he had been paid 2s 6d, a sum which had been gradually increased over the years. His conclusion was that it paid to give 'steady, careful, honest attention' to sick members and also to ask for additional payment as one felt justified. He had found on requesting a rise that his services were sufficiently valued (*Lancet*, 21 July 1877, pp. 109–10). Doctors in other localities had similar experiences (*Lancet*, 29 September 1877, p. 481). As the number of clubs paying 5s or more increased, more and more doctors concluded that it was only 'unworthy competition' that held down rates (*Lancet*, 1877, vol. 2, p. 670).

During the 1870s fees were increasing steadily. But doctors were rarely successful in securing agreement to wage limits. Very few friendly societies would agree to such a restriction on their membership. For many of them it infringed the principle that all joined on equal terms.

There were two kinds of wealthy member. There were some wealthy members, particularly farmers, who joined as honorary members – enjoying no benefit except medical attendance. In one area near Stafford, honorary members paid 9s 6d per year to the club, 3s went to the doctor, 2s 6d for the annual dinner, and the remainder was a donation to club funds (*Lancet*, 20 August 1870, pp. 278–9; 1 October 1870, p. 492). The secretary of the Weston-on-Trent Oddfellows explained the view of the friendly societies to *Lancet* readers. The societies tried to attract wealthier members as honorary members because their contributions helped the poorer brothers. The societies saw it as voluntary redistribution of income. As the secretary of one Foresters' court put it, the 5s paid by his honorary members came to £7 a year, enough to make extra Christmas payments of 7s 6d to fourteen distressed or elderly members and 2s 6d to fourteen widows (*Foresters Miscellany*, April 1885, p. 385). The doctors, however, saw this redistribution as imposing unreasonably on them, for the bait for the wealthy honorary members was medical attendance at fees lower than those the doctors had laid down for wealthier persons (*Lancet*, 17 September 1870, p. 422).

But by far the most common reason why clubs had wealthy members was that men had joined when young and lived successful lives, with the result that by middle age they were relatively well off. Such men invariably held honoured positions within the friendly societies and often chose not to give up their society membership. The feeling of the friendly societies was that these men had paid their 'medical pence' throughout their lives, and invariably made few demands on the doctor's time. Their lifetime's contributions entitled them to medical attendance whatever their later income.

The Rise of the Medical Institutes

One side-effect of the agitation of the 1860s and 1870s was the foundation of friendly society medical institutes. The first of these was opened in Preston in 1870 in response to the local doctors' campaign for an increase in medical fees. The doctors were pressing for a 50 per cent increase to a minimum of 3s 0d per annum, plus an additional mileage allowance for patients who lived outside the borough. In December 1869 the Preston friendly societies had met to consider their response to the demands of what they called the 'Preston Medical Trades Union'. The result was the foundation of the Preston Associated

Friendly Societies' Provident Dispensary in January 1870. The majority of contributors were existing friendly society members, but non-members could also join for an additional 1s 2d per quarter (*BMJ*, 23 October 1869, p. 449; 27 November 1869, p. 600; *Lancet*, 11 December 1869, p. 831).

The Preston medical institute was soon followed by others. In 1870 the Worcester Associated Friendly Societies' Medical Association was founded. And by 1874 Manchester Unity lodges had established medical institutes at Newport and Bradford (RCFS, Reports of the Assistant Commissioners, *Mr Stanley's Report*, 1874, pp. 109, 191, 206–7).

The immediate cause of the foundation of the medical institutes was the campaign of the doctors for increased fees. The underlying reason was not a wish to avoid paying more for medical care, but rather a sense of dissatisfaction with traditional lodge practice. There were three main criticisms of the traditional lodge system. First, lodge doctors were usually part-time, serving not only other friendly society branches but also taking private patients on a fee-for-service basis. Some friendly society members in certain localities felt that their lodge medical officers were more interested in building up a lucrative private practice than in serving lodge members. To secure the undivided attention of the doctor the friendly society medical institutes employed full-time salaried medical officers who were forbidden to take private patients.

The second criticism was that whilst some doctors would *prescribe* very expensive medicines, they would seldom *supply* them, preferring to advise the patient to pay extra at the chemists. Such doctors argued that the fixed annual capitation fee did not cover unusually expensive medicines. This practice was far from universal, but it did happen. The medical institutes overcame it by buying their own drugs at wholesale prices and supplying them direct in their own dispensaries. Moreover, medical institutes would also supply items such as cod liver oil, malt and other nutritional items, a lack of which was often at the root of many medical problems.

The third criticism was that lodge practice did not usually provide for dependants. The medical institutes provided for the whole family and not only the club member. In the 1870s most institutes charged 8s 0d per year for the whole family, compared with 3s 6d or 4s 0d in lodge practice for the man only. Women were attended during their confinement at the concessional rate of 10s 6d. In addition, widows and orphans of dead members were allowed to continue their membership, and in some cases orphans were attended free of charge until they reached working age.

By 1877 efforts were being made to establish medical institutes, or medical aid associations, throughout England. They had been founded in Preston, Newport, Derby, Worcester, Nottingham, Bradford and elsewhere (*Oddfellows Magazine*, October 1877, pp. 241–3). For some friendly society leaders the foundation of the medical institutes was another step in the great friendly society crusade, summed up in a phrase subsequently purloined by the welfare state: to provide for members from 'the cradle to the grave'. Leaders of the movement, it was said, would not consider their work complete until this had been achieved (*Lancet*, 26 October 1895, pp. 1070–71).

Some institutes employed one doctor, some two or more, and most took on a full-time dispenser. In the 1870s medical officers were paid about £200 a year, with their rent and rates and some other expenses thrown in. The medical institutes challenged the claim that good doctors could not be obtained at that price. They pointed out that there were many doctors who came from humble origins who, therefore, could neither buy a practice nor find friends in high places to obtain one for them. As a result their only opening was to work as an assistant to an established doctor, usually for a salary well below medical institute rates. Such men, it was said, were 'hailing with joy' the establishment of medical institutes, as these offered them their only chance of independence.

The *Lancet* consistently opposed the establishment of medical institutes. But professional opposition met with little success, and it was during this period that doctors complained of a sense of 'political powerlessness' (*Lancet*, 1883, vol. 2, p. 25; 1882, vol. 2, p. 502). One reason for the failure of professional opposition was, as we have seen, that not all doctors disliked the medical institutes. Some institute medical officers complained about conditions, whilst others were satisfied (*Lancet*, 1886, vol. 1, p. 384). One doctor, for example, described his position at a medical institute as a 'very pleasant and comfortable berth'. He claimed that the greater evil was the wealthy doctor earning £1,000 a year who took on an assistant at £60 to £80 to do much of the hard work. The assistants, who were often as well qualified as their masters, had more to put up with, he thought, than medical institute doctors (*Lancet*, 1887, vol. 1, p. 809).

This particular medical officer had about 2,500 patients. In subsequent issues of the *Lancet* some institute medical officers pointed out that they had about 4,000 patients. This number of patients, they said, produced an intolerable workload. Other doctors objected not only to the number of patients they had to attend, but to consumer control itself. Some particularly resented control by 'working men' (*Lancet*, 30 January 1886, p. 235; 27 February 1886, p. 431).

This is how one dissatisfied doctor described his conditions. He was on call seven days a week and got Christmas Day and Good Friday off only 'if nothing happened'. In addition to home visits, he would often see a hundred patients a day at the surgery, occasionally more. The family rate was 4s, with an extra sum payable for confinements. The resident medical officer was paid £180 and the non-resident £120. The former had an additional allowance for coal, gas, cleaning etc. He thought he would be three times better off if institute members came to him as ordinary club patients (*Lancet*, 1887, vol. 1, p. 340; 1887, vol. 1, p. 903; *Lancet*, 7 December 1889, p. 1209).

The institutes also had their critics within the friendly societies. Some were criticized for excessive emphasis on cheapness. Doctors who would accept low salaries, it was claimed by one friendly society leader, were men who 'cannot mend themselves' or those who were constantly on the lookout for something better (*Foresters Miscellany*, April 1884, p. 87). Some of the institutes, managed by working men with little to call their own and accustomed to 'scrimping and saving' to make ends meet, certainly paid low salaries; but most soon learned that in medicine, as in other walks of life, cheapness did not always mean good value.

Among the early medical institutes was the York Friendly Societies' Medical Association, founded in 1877. It was governed by a general committee made up of one delegate for every hundred (or part of a hundred) members in each affiliated society or branch. A committee of management carried out day-today administration. In 1877 the capitation fee was 3s per member, plus a 1s entrance fee. The medical officers' hours were typical of other institutes. They were required to attend on weekdays from 9–10 a.m., 2–3 p.m., and 6–8 p.m., and on Sundays from 9–10 a.m. Home visits were to be made in the remainder of the time: 'They shall prescribe for and supply the best medical treatment in their power to all sick patients, and they shall visit when necessary all patients unable to attend the Dispensary. . .' To ensure that medical officers devoted their energies wholeheartedly to members, private practice was forbidden.

The Bradford FSMA had been established in 1872. Relations with their medical officer in the 1880s seem to have been good. In the annual report for 1888 the management committee wrote:

> It is a pleasing duty to have to report that universal satisfaction prevails amongst our members at the manner in which our Medical Officer, Mr Michael Hayes, performs his duties, more especially by those who, unfortunately, have required his valuable professional aid during sickness; his kindly disposition, untiring energy, great professional ability, and a constant devotedness to the welfare of our members, have secured for him the gratitude and esteem of all those whom he has had the opportunity of meeting.

And in his own report the medical officer said: 'Allow me once more to offer you and the members of the Association generally my very hearty thanks for your many acts of kindness to me during the time I have been your medical officer and to wish you one and all a long run of prosperity and happiness in the brighter days that seem to be dawning on our valuable institution.' Obviously it was customary to exchange courtesies in annual reports, but these sentiments seem to go beyond the normal requirement.

This doctor seems to have been well paid, receiving £353 3s 0d, out of which he had to pay a dispenser (who would have earned £60 to £80 a year). The association provided him with a house rent-free, gas, coal, a stable, two horses, a groom, and a trap, all of which were valued at £253 in 1888. Membership in 1888 was 3,380, involving the medical officer in 8,287 home visits, dispensing 23,317 prescriptions, and attending twenty-eight confinements. He also examined 400 candidates for admission to lodges. If his visits were carried out over six days, this works out at twenty-six home visits a day.

In 1879 the Friendly Societies Medical Alliance (FSMA) had been established to promote the common interests of friendly society medical institutes. By 1882 the FSMA had established a medical agency (a kind of labour exchange) at which doctors deposited their names and qualifications and to which medical institutes turned when they needed a doctor (*Foresters Miscellany*, April 1884, pp. 86–7). In 1883, thirty-two medical institutes with a total of 139,000 members sent full returns to the FSMA. There were institutes in Bradford, Birmingham, Bristol, Derby, Exeter, Greenock, Hull, Hartlepool, Leeds, Leicester, Lincoln, Lowestoft, Newport, Northampton, Portsmouth, Reading, Sheffield, West Bromwich, Wolverhampton, and elsewhere. The largest was at York, with 9,300 members. Two years later there were forty-two medical institutes affiliated to the FSMA, with a total of 211,000 members (*Foresters Miscellany*, April 1884, p. 89; 1886, p. 145).

In 1898 there were about forty medical institutes registered as friendly societies with around 213,000 members, employing about seventy-five medical officers. In addition there were unregistered medical institutes. In 1896 there were at least five with around 19,000 members (*Foresters Directory*, 1896, pp. 593–6; *BMJ*, 10 June 1899, p. 1413). At least twenty owned their own premises, combining surgery, dispensary, and doctor's living accomodation. Annual capitation fees varied, but were usually 3s for men, 4s to 5s for wives, and 1s for children. In some cases an inclusive fee for the whole family was charged, varying from 3s 6d to around 8s 0d. The fee for confinements remained at 10s 6d. The largest institute was at Derby with 11,600 members. York was the second largest with 10,300 members, followed by Wolverhampton with 8,700 (*Foresters Directory*, 1896).

The medical institutes were proud of their self-governing character. According to W.H. Young, a friendly society leader from Kidderminster, the medical institutes represented the 'independent spirit' which was 'so necessary to the well-being of every institution, especially those relating to the working classes'. By organizing their own medical care they had freed themselves from the attentions of unsatisfactory club doctors, caricatured as offering only coloured water for medicine: 'They are no longer under that despotic system from which sprang the ever-lasting "magenta and water" which did them no earthly good, and from whence also they were continually hearing the remark, "what can you expect for a penny a week"' (*Foresters Miscellany*, April 1881, pp. 400–401).

This pride in their autonomy continued to be part of the make-up of the medical institutes. The preface to the 1896 rules of the Luton Friendly Societies Medical Institute stated its objectives: to provide professional attendance and the 'best' of medicines by the payment of annual contributions, 'thus obviating the necessity of appealing to any charity . . . and relieving our members from the fear of the "doctor's bill" which inevitably follows the advice or attendance of a medical practitioner in private practice.'

The institute, the preface said, 'is managed by *working men*, who should best understand their own wants and how to meet them' (emphasis in the original). The writer complained that in the beginning their aims had been 'grossly misrepresented' by the medical profession, but gradually their membership had expanded. In January 1889 they had begun with 1,500 members. Soon this had climbed to 5,500. The Luton Friendly Societies Medical Institute had been established in January 1889, and functioned until it was dissolved in 1948 as a result of the foundation of the NHS. By the turn of the century it was probably the finest of all the medical institutes, a fact later to be of importance during the Parliamentary debate on the 1911 National Insurance Act.

Some medical institutes opened branches to add to the convenience of members. In 1907 the Leeds FSMA operated from two buildings, with a dispensary and full-time resident medical officer at each. Membership was around 8,000. The original Sheffield medical institute had been wound up by 1907 and a new one established which operated from three separate dispensaries in order to reduce members' travelling (RCPL, 1909, Appendix IV, Q. 41489(18), Appendix LXXX, Q. 42262(8,9)).

Growing Professional Militancy
Many doctors were satisfied with the results of the late 1860s and early 1870s agitation, but by the 1880s complaints were being voiced with renewed vigour (see e.g. *BMJ*, 6 March 1880, p.

389). In some areas in the 1880s there were good feelings between doctors and the lodges (e.g. *Lancet*, 5 November 1887, p.
936). But in other localities doctors signed pledges not to work
for the lodges (*Lancet*, 5 October 1889, p. 720).

However it was not till the 1890s that pressure began to mount
for a more concerted approach. Doctors were still complaining
about low fees and about wealthy club patients. But there were
lesser complaints too. Some doctors expressed their hostility to
contract practice in terms of hostility to 'trade' or trading
methods. This had partly to do with aristocratic hostility to those
who had to earn their living, but was chiefly a disguised hostility
to competition. The specific targets of doctors who condemned
trade were not payment as such, but advertising and canvassing.
Such methods smacked of the 'costermonger-physic' (*BMJ*, 10
October 1896, p. 1067). Doctors did not object to the selling of
practices or to charging ordinary fees on the ground that these
smacked of 'trade'. They only complained when competition
left them worse off financially than they desired.

Some doctors complained about the extension of contract
practice to women and children. According to the *Lancet* special
commissioner, one of the attractions of club practice was that
although the man of the family had to be attended for the capitation rate, the wife and children would also use the doctor and
pay the ordinary fee. When moves began to be made for contract practice to be extended to the whole family, doctors who
looked upon it as a useful 'introduction' to the family became
worried that they would be financially worse off. By the mid
1890s more and more friendly societies were seeking to extend
ordinary contract practice to wives and children. In Great Yarmouth, where doctors were well organized, they complained
about the opening of special juvenile clubs, the emergence of
medical aid associations for wives and children, the opening of a
Female Foresters club; and the growing tendency to admit the
well-to-do (*BMJ*, 7 November 1896, p. 1408). Doctors feared
that these developments would lead to the virtual disappearance
of private practice. As a result many refused to accept women as
contract patients.

In other respects, the rules governing contract practice were
sometimes becoming more burdensome. For example, one
court of the Ancient Order of Foresters imposed a new rule on

its medical officer which required him to pay the complainant's expenses if a charge of 'neglect' was proved against him (*BMJ*, 26 December 1896, p. 1848). Doctors also complained that they were often expected to perform operations free of charge (*BMJ*, 8 February 1896, p. 368).

By the end of 1895 the *Lancet* was urging, indeed it 'expected', every doctor to join in the battle of the clubs to put right the profession's grievances (*Lancet*, 28 December 1895, pp. 1647–8). Yarmouth doctors were in the forefront of the battle and established a trade combination. They approached the local benefit societies demanding new terms. In October 1896 local societies reacted angrily and asked the doctors to pledge themselves not to raise their demands again. The doctors declined and the societies advertised successfully for alternative practitioners (*Lancet*, 24 February 1900, p. 577). As we have seen, some medical institutes were established as an act of retaliation against professional combinations. The Wigan friendly societies for example, retaliated against the *BMJ* warning notice by founding a medical hall (*BMJ*, 22 December 1900, p. 1814). Yarmouth friendly societies responded similarly to a combination of Yarmouth's doctors. They established the Amalgamated Friendly Societies Medical Institute, which was promptly boycotted by local doctors in January 1897. There were two medical institute doctors, but the other seventeen Yarmouth doctors did succeed – after coercing one reluctant colleague into joining them – in totally isolating them. However, when specialist assistance was required the institute sent patients to London (*Lancet*, 3 March 1900, pp. 655–7). The foundation of the institute proved very costly to the Yarmouth doctors. It was estimated that it cost them about £2,000 a year in lost club contributions (*Oddfellows Magazine*, February 1897, p. 42). One of their leaders was James Smith Whittaker. In 1902 he became the first Medical Secretary of the BMA, whereupon he devoted much of his energy to the destruction of contract practice. In 1911 the government appointed him a member of the joint insurance committee and the English insurance commission, a position which enabled him to stifle the growth of the medical institutes (see below). Later he became Senior Medical Officer in the Ministry of Health.

Doctors in other parts of the country met with as little success as the Yarmouth doctors. One doctor practising in Scotland reported to the 1905 inquiry how doctors in his locality had made a joint demand for an increase from 2s 6d to 3s 0d. The demand was refused and the thirteen friendly societies agreed to amalgamate in a Friendly Societies' Council to advertise for outside doctors. They got 'numerous applications and had not the slightest difficulty in getting a medical officer'. Local doctors were 'hopelessly defeated' (BMA, CPR, p. 54).

Doctors in Stafford met a similar response. A meeting was held between local doctors and friendly society delegates. The doctors asked for 5s in place of the existing 4s rate; the same rate for children; and an examination fee of 2s 6d instead of 1s. They presented the friendly societies with an ultimatum: only on these terms would they either accept new appointments or continue in their existing ones. The delegates rejected the proposed increase but suggested an increase in juvenile rates from 2s 6d to 3s. A further resolution was carried that if the doctors insisted on resigning a full-time salaried doctor should be appointed under the control of the Friendly Societies Committee (*BMJ*, 1 February 1896, p. 288).

Lowest Fee Not Always Sought

But it was not everywhere that the friendly societies reacted in this manner. The local combination of doctors in Portsmouth, the Portsmouth Medical Union, met a variety of responses. These serve to remind us of the diversity that is possible within a free market, and as a warning against over-simple generalization about free markets – over-simplifications to which many modern scholars seem particularly prone. Professor Bently Gilbert, for example, cites the assertion of Alfred Cox that 'it was no secret that many of the appointments were obtained by bribery and corruption'. And Gilbert continues, 'Jobs were auctioned off to the lowest bidder' (1966, p. 309). Even Professor Klein has succumbed. The societies were intent on 'cutting to the bone' the annual fee to doctors. The customer, he comments, 'was always right – but the customer insisted on cheap medicine' (Klein, 1973, p. 63).

In addition to seeking pay increases from friendly societies, medical aid societies and Poor Law Guardians, the Portsmouth Medical Union set out to maintain a 'patients black list'. Doctors also sought to prevent the extension of contract practice to women (*Lancet*, 21 September 1895, p. 757; *BMJ*, 15 June 1895, p. 1342; *BMJ*, 26 October 1895, p. 1053). Their campaign for higher fees met a mixed response.

The two medical officers of the Portsmouth Medical Benefit Society, a society run by dockyard workers and funded by pay-packet deductions, resigned in protest at the low fees. The dock workers found other doctors to fill their places. However, some dock workers sympathized with the original medical officers and established a new benefit society which offered them more favourable terms (*Lancet*, 21 September 1895, p. 757). A couple of months later, in November 1895, elections to one of Portsmouth's largest Oddfellows lodges were held. The existing medical officer, Dr Lord, was refusing to accept the new terms on offer, and specifically juvenile rates of 2s 6d per annum for children aged between three months and fifteen years. Dr Lord demanded 4s per annum. Three outside competitors stood against him, much to the chagrin of the *BMJ*. One offered to attend juveniles at 2s 6d, one at 2s and another at 1s 6d. In the event Dr Lord was so well respected that he was decisively re-elected at his higher fee, having won 168 votes against 65, 31 and 11 for his opponents (*BMJ*, 23 November 1895, p. 1319; *BMJ*, 30 November 1895, p. 1368). Another doctor reported a similar experience to the *BMJ* inquiry: 'The society I am medical officer to were asked by a rival practitioner to transfer their work to him for an average price of 1s 6d per head per annum.' But, he said, 'They remained steadfast to me. . .' (BMA, CPR, 1905, p. 45).

Around the same time the Rechabites in Portsmouth elected their surgeon. The sitting surgeon had demanded 4s and was opposed by candidates offering to serve for 3s 6d and 3s. The sitting candidate was not re-elected, but they did not appoint the cheapest doctor. The candidate who tendered 3s 6d was elected (*BMJ*, 12 September 1896, p. 684).

Elsewhere, we also find a mixed picture. In one case a doctor's resignation was met by an appeal from an Oddfellows' lodge to come back on better terms (*BMJ*, 3 March 1900, p. 556). By contrast, doctors in Cowes tried to organize against the friendly societies, but were defeated. The leading doctor in the conflict lost most of his income (*Lancet*, 7 April 1900, pp. 1031–3). In Stockport a meeting was called to vote on an increase from

2s 6d to 3s 6d. The increase was rejected by a large majority (*BMJ*, 14 March 1896, p. 672). Some doctors objected to the requirement that they should become honorary members of the society which employed them, but found they could not even secure this modest concession. One doctor complained of his treatment by the Hand-in-Hand Benefit Society in Guildford. When he declined to join the society he was sacked (*Lancet*, 3 March 1900, p. 654). On some occasions low fee levels obtained even though the friendly societies were quite willing to pay more. Fees of, say, 5s were accepted by both friendly societies and local doctors but along came new doctors volunteering to work for less. The editor of the *BMJ* attacked colleagues who practised such 'disloyalty'. He knew of 'several instances' of 5s fees being agreed, only for the agreement to be undermined by doctors, one by one, accepting 4s or even 3s (*BMJ*, 1900, vol. 2, p. 1039).

In the 1890s the campaigns against the clubs had begun to be more effectively organized. By 1895 the *Lancet* had appointed a special commissioner to report on 'the battle of the clubs'. The first report was published in August 1895 and dealt with a dispute in Brussels. Reports on the situation in Britain soon followed and by December 1896, thirty-seven reports had been published. From 1895 the *BMJ* index carried regular references to the battle of the clubs. By 1896 calls were being made to adopt an openly trade union stance. And some doctors were condemning their less militant colleagues as 'blacklegs' (*BMJ*, 1896, vol. 1, p. 999; vol. 2, p. 8; 1897, vol. 1, p. 168). But notwithstanding the increased organization and increased militancy of the profession, doctors' attempts to establish monopolies continued to fail. Professional efforts to raise fees met a range of responses, and capitation fees increased steadily towards 4s or 5s. But whenever a professional combination was faced with determined opposition from the friendly societies, the doctors were defeated.

What does the evidence tell us about the attitude of the consumer? Paraphrasing Professor Klein, a fair conclusion would seem to be that the customer was always right, and the customer insisted, not on cheap medicine, but on the best quality care at the price he could afford.

3

From Local Combinations to Using the Power of the State

As some doctors grew frustrated with the failure of their efforts at combination they argued that trade combination was doomed to failure. They advised recourse to a new method: more vigorous use of the powers of the General Medical Council to overcome the dominant consumer.

The Rise of the Medical Practitioner
Before considering how the medical profession attempted to use the power of the state, it will be helpful to consider the recent history of attempts by governments to regulate medical practice. In the fourteenth and fifteenth centuries physicians were usually university graduates and had a strong connection with the church. The medieval church did not approve the shedding of blood and gave no encouragement to surgery. As a result the practice of surgery evolved separately from 'physic'.

There were a number of early attempts to license the practice of physic. Henry VIII granted a charter to the Royal College of Physicians in 1518. Following the continental model, the Royal College was partly a learned academy and partly a guild. An Act of 1522 granted a monopoly on the practice of physic to those examined and approved by the Royal College or by the Universities of Oxford and Cambridge. The surgeons were much lower in status at this stage of their history, and in 1540 amalgamated with the barbers, though no barber was to practise surgery and no surgeon was to cut hair.

There was also licensing by the Church. Legislation of 1421 provided that physicians must be approved by universities and surgeons by guilds. In 1511 an Act required the examination of physicians and surgeons and forbade practice by unlicensed persons. Except for graduates of Oxford and Cambridge, candidates in London were to be examined by the Bishop of London or the Dean of St Paul's with the aid of advice from physicians, and in the country by the Bishop of the Diocese.

For many years the Royal College of Physicians did much to advance medical knowledge, but by the end of the seventeenth century it had lost its commitment to medical advance, and its affairs were being conducted purely in the interests of its members. Membership was severely curtailed. One result of this abuse was the rise of the apothecaries. They began as a type of grocer. In a charter of 1606, granted to grocers, apothecaries were specifically mentioned. In 1617 apothecaries received a separate charter, and grocers were forbidden to sell drugs. The Society of Apothecaries claimed an ancient right both to prescribe and to supply medicines.

By the late seventeenth century both the Royal College of Physicians and the Barber-Surgeons Company were tending to act in a purely selfish spirit. The great mass of people had no alternative but to turn to the apothecaries. The Royal College was not unaware of the danger of this competition and one result was that in 1687 it ruled that its members should offer free medicine in certain circumstances. As a result a free dispensary was opened in 1688. Others followed. But for the most part the Royal College showed little interest in providing for the general population. In 1703, in an important case, the House of Lords ruled that apothecaries could prescribe medicines and recommend treatment, as well as dispense drugs. As a result apothecaries continued to develop as medical practitioners. An Act of 1748 allowed the Society of Apothecaries to issue licences without which no one could dispense medicine in London.

During the seventeenth century the surgeons were held in check by the Bishops, who controlled the licensing system. But during the eighteenth century their knowledge and skill was expanding steadily and in 1745 surgeons separated from the Barber-Surgeons Company to become the Company of Surgeons. In 1800 the Royal College of Surgeons of London was granted a charter in the place of the Company of Surgeons. (The college was to become the Royal College of Surgeons of England in 1843.)

By the late eighteenth century it was becoming common for apothecaries to train as surgeons. Then in 1815 the Apothecaries Act gave the Society of Apothecaries the power to examine all apothecaries in England and Wales. The apothecaries put the Act to beneficial use. A five-year apprenticeship was prescribed and no one was allowed to practise without a licence. Chemists and druggists in existence at the time of the Act were, however, allowed to continue to trade. The Society of Apothecaries introduced written examinations and tightened up the licensing system. Soon after 1815 private medical schools opened up, and later hospital medical schools emerged, University College being the first in 1827. Most licentiates of the Society of Apothecaries were also licensed by the Royal College of Surgeons and by 1830 it had become common to call anyone so licensed a general practitioner (Carr-Saunders & Wilson, 1933).

The Act of 1815 succeeded in providing a framework which permitted the emergence of a class of trained general practitioners. But it had also been hoped that the unqualified would be eliminated. This had not occurred. By 1830 there were eighteen licensing authorities and the GPs were still being looked upon as inferiors by the physicians. A movement developed for a single licensing authority. A Select Committee was appointed in 1834 and there was virtually constant agitation until the Act of 1858.

This created the General Medical Council, not in place of the existing licensing authorities, but above them. Initially it had twenty-three members, nine nominated by the medical corporations, eight by the universities, and six by the Crown. In 1886 the Crown representatives were reduced to five, and five more were added, elected by the general body of practitioners. Usually the successful candidates were those who enjoyed the support of the BMA. Over the years new universities have also been given representation.

The GMC was required to register persons who could produce a licence and pay the fee. They could, however, remove a doctor from the register on certain grounds. But the GMC neither taught nor examined. It had no direct power over licensing authorities, but if it disapproved of one it could make representations to the Privy Council which could withdraw its power to issue licences. From 1884 the Royal College of Physicians and the Royal College of Surgeons had examined jointly. And in 1886 an Act required that qualifications must be in both medicine and surgery, thus formally ending the separate development of physic and surgery.

The State as a Regulator

In the 1890s doctors began, in a repetition of past abuses of state power, to try to put the powers of the GMC to work in service of their pecuniary interests. The chief attraction of the General Medical Council was that it had the power to remove doctors from the medical register, which effectively meant to put them out of business. It could do so on two main grounds: (a) if they were guilty of a felony or a misdemeanour; or (b) if they were guilty of 'infamous conduct in any professional respect'. There was no appeal against its decisions.

The Medical Act of 1858, section 29, empowered the General Medical Council as follows:

If any registered medical practitioner . . . shall after due inquiry be judged by the General Council to have been guilty of infamous conduct in any professional respect, the General Council may if they see fit direct the Registrar to erase the name of such medical practitioner from the *Register*.

The power was tempered by section 52:

Provided always that nothing herein contained shall extend to authorise Her Majesty to create any new restriction in the practice of medicine or surgery, or to grant to any of the said corporations any powers or privileges contrary to the common law of the land.

Some doctors took the view that it constituted infamous conduct to fail to cooperate with professional restrictive practices intended to limit competition and raise fees. These doctors tried to use the General Medical Council to get other colleagues struck off the Medical Register for failing to engage in such restrictive trade practices. These moves began in earnest in 1892.

The approach to the GMC was led by the Medical Defence Union (MDU) and took the form of an attack on medical aid associations, a term which included commercial medical aid companies, as well as non-profit medical aid societies, provident dispensaries and friendly society medical institutes. The *British Medical Journal* supported the MDU, arguing that medical association doctors were 'practically "sweated"' for the profit of the associations. The *BMJ* wanted the GMC to declare employment by a medical aid association 'professionally degrading'.

In their anxiety to find grounds which would permit the GMC to act the MDU tried to draw an analogy with an earlier GMC ruling on covering for unqualified persons. The GMC had ruled that for a registered practitioner to act as the cover for an unqualified person in order that the unqualified individual could carry on medical practice as if he were qualified was 'infamous conduct in a professional respect', within the meaning of section 29 of the 1858 Act. The MDU argued that medical aid association doctors were covering in exactly the same way for the medical aid association committee. Even the *BMJ*, however, pointed out that there was a very clear distinction (*BMJ*, 15 October 1892, p. 854). The GMC's response was to appoint a committee which reported in June 1893.

The criticisms of the MDU were answered by a doctor serving as the medical officer of a friendly society medical institute. He refuted the view that medical officers were 'sweated', and argued that, on the contrary, they had taken positions as medical officers to escape previous sweating practised on them by other doctors who had employed them as assistants. He pointed out that all his colleagues had had to work harder for less pay as assistants to private practitioners than they did for medical institutes. Most had been given workloads at least twice as heavy while they were assistants, and some had carried burdens three times as great. Indeed, this was a long-standing grievance (e.g. *Association Medical Journal*, 7 October 1853, p. 888). He denied that the friendly societies made profits from their work. If there was a surplus, as there occasionally was, it was re-invested to provide security of incomes in the future: 'We are quite satisfied that our income should be thus secured, and we do not lay claim to this money' (*BMJ*, 22 October 1892, p. 920).

His view was supported by a doctor from South Wales who pointed out that he received better pay from the 'Medical Aid' than he would have from the miners' club – the main local alternative – which was based on pay-packet deductions (*BMJ*, 22

October 1892, p. 370). Another medical officer of a medical aid association pointed out that if there was no association he would end up treating many of his patients under the Poor Law for much less (*BMJ*, 5 November 1892, p. 1028). Several other doctors, however, wrote to the *BMJ* criticizing medical aid associations, including one who described himself as 'another MO of friendly societies' (*BMJ*, 29 October 1892, pp. 970–1; *BMJ*, 5 November 1892, pp. 1027–8; see also *BMJ*, 12 November 1892, p. 1067).

A conference of twenty-one friendly societies memorialized the General Medical Council in March 1893 emphasizing that friendly society medical institutes could not be described as organizations for the profit of their promoters and that they provided a service by mutual aid (*Oddfellows Magazine*, 1893, p. 134). Simultaneously a leading article in the *Oddfellows Magazine* pointed out that there was no objection to doctors' combinations which sought to enforce a minimum wage. But it was a very different matter to try to deny some doctors the choice of working for a medical aid association, or indeed to deny a doctor the right to work for whoever he pleased (*Oddfellows Magazine*, March 1893, p. 69). The friendly societies felt that the attempt to use the power of the state (exercised by the GMC) represented an attempt to combine for improper ends. To try to raise wages by combination they believed to be legitimate; but to attempt to deny other doctors the right to work for the friendly societies was wholly illegitimate.

The GMC committee believed there were about sixty medical aid associations, including those run by insurance companies. It surveyed all their medical officers. In 1891 the FSMA had fifty-one affiliated associations, but it is not clear how many of these are included in the survey findings. The GMC committee received eighty-five answers to their eleven-point questionnaire. In answer to the question, 'Is the amount of work imposed on you such as to permit you conscientiously to give the necessary amount of attention to individual cases?', forty-five answered 'yes' and thirty-three, 'no'. On the question of profits the committee concluded that 'on the whole it cannot be said that the profits . . . are at all great' (GMC, 1893, p. 14).

Medical officers did feel, in the ratio of fifty-five to twenty-nine, that some of their patients could have afforded to pay higher fees. About half of the respondents were forbidden to engage in private practice, and half were not. Forty-nine reported that no canvassing was used, and twenty-six that their association did canvass (*BMJ*, 3 June 1893, p. 1168). The medical aid departments run by insurance companies went in for canvassing on a large scale, and the medical institutes of the friendly societies did not. The committee was conscious of the differences between friendly society medical institutes and the commercial organizations and commented that in presenting their report they 'desired to show great deference to the legitimate and beneficial work of the friendly societies' (GMC, 1893, p. 8). They demonstrated their confidence in the Friendly Societies Medical Alliance by recommending that all medical institutes should conform to its Guide-Rules (ibid., p. 18).

Nevertheless, they criticized several friendly society medical institutes for not observing the Guide-Rules issued by the FSMA. These laid down that 2,000 patients or more required one full-time medical officer; more than 2,500 and up to no more than 3,500 required one medical officer plus a full-time dispenser; more than 3,000, and certainly more than 3,500, up to as many as 4,500 required a senior medical officer plus an assistant medical officer; more than this and certainly 5,000 plus required either three medical officers or two doctors plus a full-time dispenser. According to the GMC committee these limits were 'often exceeded'. At Northampton there were 14,369 members with three doctors, at Wolverhampton 11,000 served by two doctors, with similar ratios at Derby, Nottingham, Leicester and York. As a result few doctors held office for long. But the committee had no complaints about the standard of medicines prescribed. The institutes were 'well supplied with pure drugs' (p. 9). Medical officers asked if lay committees interfered with their decisions to issue or not issue sickness certificates. The great majority said they were free to do what they thought right. And friendly society spokesmen pointed out that it was in the societies' interests to 'uphold the perfect independence' of medical officers. However, one medical officer had been dismissed for refusing a certificate to a sick man (ibid., p. 16).

The Medical Defence Union, which had initiated the complaint, was demanding that service in a medical institute be declared infamous conduct, except where an appointment was on ordinary club terms (ibid., p. 24). The committee did not agree. In June 1893 the GMC reaffirmed an earlier ruling on covering for the unqualified, but it rejected a recommendation that a general practitioner was acting in a 'reprehensible manner' if (a) he held an appointment which meant that he could not do justice to his patients; (b) he gave certificates which were not justified on medical grounds; (c) his employing association employed canvassers. Some members of the GMC argued that it would be *ultra vires* to pass such a resolution, and others that the GMC had no power to advise doctors or to 'protect their pecuniary interests' (*BMJ*, 3 June 1893, pp. 1169–70). The GMC concluded that the investigation by their committee had not 'disclosed the prevalence of any offences with which it falls within the statutory province of the Council to deal' (*Foresters Miscellany*, August 1893, p. 142). E.M. Little, the official historian of the BMA, later attacked the GMC for having 'shirked' their responsibility in the matter (1932, p. 202).

In the mid 1890s conditions in friendly society medical institutes varied from place to place. The medical officers at Lincoln complained that the friendly societies medical institute 'sweated' them (*Lancet*, 12 October 1895, pp. 944–5; 26 October 1895, pp. 1070–71). But in the best of the institutes conditions were far from undesirable. The *Lancet* special commissioner, for example, reported very favourably on the situation in York, where doctors and the friendly societies worked harmoniously together.

Dr Ramsay, the president of the York medical society, blamed fellow members of the medical profession for causing the formation of clubs. He cited cases of bills of £15 being presented to servant girls who would have barely earned that much in a whole year. In another case a bill of £30 had been presented to a man with an annual income of £200. The York friendly societies medical institute supported three medical men who were as well off as they would have been if their club patients had been private patients paying a separate fee for each consultation. Dr Ramsay argued that these families could pay £2 to £3 a year without financial hardship, but if they were charged £5 or £10 they would probably pay nothing at all. It was preferable that they should pay from 8s to 12s a year through a friendly society. The senior medical officer to the institute told the commissioner that he was satisfied. His income was safe, it was sufficient for him to live in comfort, to bring up his family and to have some enjoyment in life. He was allowed an occasional holiday, was not overworked, and had received extra help during an influenza epidemic. The dispensary was not greatly abused by rich men. One reason perhaps, was that he insisted that everyone in the waiting room should see him in strict rotation. Few new members earned more than 25s a week, but some rose to better circumstances in later life and kept up their membership (*Lancet*, 7 December 1895, pp. 1458–9).

Pay and conditions in the medical institutes varied, but the lowest rate of pay seems to have been £120 per year for the most junior appointments. On top of this there was usually free accommodation plus heating and travel allowances. Senior medical officers usually received in excess of £200, and good men commanded well over £300. There were plenty of applicants for vacancies, even at the lowest salaries. For example, in 1893 there were seventy-five applicants for one medical aid association at a salary of £120, plus a house (*Oddfellows Magazine*, March 1893, p. 68). This was because many established doctors in private practice were employing doctors as assistants for far less, often at from £60 to £80 a year.

Some of the resentment towards medical institutes was expressed, not by serving institute medical officers, but by doctors who had lost lucrative club positions through the establishment of institutes. For example, the surgeon to the Manchester Unity lodge in Stourport was displaced by a medical institute. He felt particularly aggrieved because six years earlier he had started his own penny-a-week club for women and children and also did honorary service in a nearby infirmary. In 1889 the Stourport medical institute had a membership of nearly 3,000 out of a population of 4,500. According to the displaced doctor this was because all the well-to-do tradesmen had joined (*Oddfellows Magazine*, November 1889, p. 347). The president of the institute, however, said the main reason for its establishment had been dissatisfaction with lodge practice. Contract patients and private patients had not been treated equally. Moreover, under the medical institute scheme families were included, and medical officers prescribed the best medicines regardless of cost (*Oddfellows Magazine*, January 1890, p. 13).

Renewed Pressure on the GMC

From time to time further calls were made to declare employment by a medical aid association 'infamous conduct' under section 29. In 1896, even the *BMJ* were unwilling to endorse this view without further consideration, although they favoured some kind of GMC ruling (*BMJ*, 15 February 1896, p. 435). However, a further attempt to use the power of the General Medical Council was made in 1897 when Norwich doctors put forward a new proposal. The same doctors also tried (unsuccessfully) to persuade the Royal College of Surgeons and the Royal College of Physicians to forbid their members from accepting positions in medical institutes (*BMJ*, 24 July 1897, p. 238).

The Norwich FSMI had been established in 1872 and by 1897 had over 10,000 members. There were two full-time salaried medical officers, a consulting physician and a consulting surgeon, though the consultants had just been successfully put under pressure to resign. The complaint of the Norwich doctors was that the FSMI was a 'trading society conducted by laymen' for medical attendance. The annual subscription of 3s was not all passed on to the medical officers. Instead it was used to pay working expenses and to improve the premises (GMC, *Minutes*, 1897, pp. 201–2). The response of the GMC was to appoint a committee which did not report in full until June 1899. The delay was due to a long inquiry into the cause of the friction between the profession and medical aid associations. Two meetings with the friendly societies had been held and two main problems identified. The first was that the remuneration was too low, particularly because women and children were now being included in contract practice when hitherto they had usually been excluded. The second was that some clubs had wealthy members who could pay higher fees.

The committee recommended the establishment of a conciliation board to resolve the differences with the friendly societies. The representatives of the friendly societies, they believed, were as anxious as the profession to terminate the friction between them. The committee drew a sharp distinction between the friendly societies' medical institutes, whose members belonged to 'the industrial classes' and who did not employ paid canvassers, and the medical aid societies run by the insurance companies, in which medical attendance was thrown in as bait for life assurance business. In these cases it was believed that wholesale 'canvassing and touting' was practised. Medical institutes, said the report, 'composed of *bona fide* members of friendly societies, and managed on sound principles, are entitled to, and have always received, the friendly consideration of the medical profession.' The friendly societies' representatives they had met had shown a strong desire to ascertain the views of the profession and to entertain the views of the GMC committee (GMC, *Minutes*, 1898, pp. 91–2, 206).

At that stage doctors were directing their most vehement criticism at the commercial medical aid companies, run largely by insurance companies. No doctor, it was felt by some colleagues, should be 'the stalking horse' of these companies (*BMJ*, 15 February 1896 p. 434). In the view of the *BMJ* it was 'degrading to any medical man to allow his professional knowledge to be used by a commercial company as its stock-in-trade' from which a profit was to be derived. On this there was to be 'no compromise'. Fair remuneration, however, was a different matter. It was not a question of principle, but a matter in which a balance must be struck between the parties (*BMJ*, 22 May 1897, p. 1302).

The committee of the GMC recommended that its parent body 'strongly disapprove' of medical practitioners who associated with medical aid associations which systematically canvassed and advertised for the purpose of procuring patients. The GMC unanimously resolved in favour of this resolution (GMC, *Minutes*, 1899, p. 177). However, this still fell short of ruling that employment by a medical aid society was 'infamous conduct'. The committee made it clear that this resolution only applied to companies canvassing and advertising to push insurance business intended to yield a profit (ibid., p. 532).

Some commercial medical aid companies stopped taking new patients at this time. The London and Manchester Industrial Assurance Company, which had 1,000 doctors under contract, told the GMC that its medical aid department had stopped taking new patients. They also vigorously denied that the department had ever been a source of profit (GMC, *Minutes*, 1899, p. 177).

Although the GMC's hostility to canvassing and advertising was confined to the use of such methods by commercial companies, within the profession generally there were many who applied no such limitation. Their intention was to stamp out all competition by force as this resolution passed in July 1899 by the County of Durham Medical Union shows:

That when the Qualified Practitioners of any district make a combined effort to raise the standard of their fees, and thereby the status of the profession, it should be deemed infamous conduct in a professional respect for any Registered Practitioner to attempt to frustrate their efforts by opposing them at cheaper rates of payment, and canvassing for patients. . .

The union explained to the GMC that they had been trying to raise contract medical fees in mining districts from 6d per fortnight to 9d. In some areas miners had refused the increase and established medical associations to employ doctors at a salary. These associations collected subscriptions and canvassed for patients. If it was not 'illegal', the union told the GMC, then they certainly thought it was 'scandalous' (GMC, *Minutes*, 1899, p. 275).

Many doctors resented the GMC's refusal to intervene. One Rotherham doctor, who believed it was useless to go in for local combinations, because these always broke down through fear of outside doctors coming in, strongly criticized the General Medical Council. He argued that, as things stood, the GMC was 'absolutely useless' to general practitioners. The GMC held that it had no power to regulate the terms on which doctors were employed. This, he argued, was because its members were professors and consultants and not affected financially by contract practice. If the GMC were composed of a 'preponderance' of GPs he felt 'it would soon discover' that it had the power to deal with contract practice (*BMJ*, 3 March 1900, p. 546).

The medical aid associations committee reported to the GMC again in December 1900. The GMC re-affirmed its earlier view that a conciliation board should be established to resolve the differences with the friendly societies, despite the lack of enthusiasm from the BMA. The majority of the GMC held to its principled line that the resolution of these 'trade' problems was not a matter for the GMC but for the profession itself, acting through the BMA (*BMJ*, 15 December 1900, pp. 1720–21). The National Conference of Friendly Societies continued to appoint delegates to this conciliation board for some years, but largely because the BMA persisted in dragging its feet the conciliation board never met. In 1901 the BMA did appoint a committee to 'watch progress in a spirit favourable to the formation' of a conciliation board. But the chief stumbling block was the BMA's insistence on the acceptance of a wage limit to exclude higher-paid workers as a pre-condition of their attendance of conciliation board meetings. The friendly societies declined to accept this condition (RFS, *Annual Report*, 1901; GMC, *Minutes*, 1901, p. 85).

Pressure on the General Medical Council was maintained. Some doctors were openly arguing for it to be used to enforce specific rates of pay. One doctor, for example, complained of the 'beggarly pittance' which contract practice afforded, and called on the GMC to rule it 'infamous conduct' to accept less than a minimum fee (*BMJ*, 24 March 1900, p. 739). The more vigorous use of the 'infamous conduct' power was again proposed to the GMC but got little support. In 1900, a resolution that association with medical aid societies and clubs which systematically canvass for patients may be regarded by the Council as 'infamous conduct in a professional respect, rendering any practitioner proved to be guilty thereof liable to have his name removed from the Medical Register' was withdrawn for the time being (*BMJ*, 15 December 1900, pp. 1720–21).

At times, to the regret of some of its members, meetings of the GMC came close to tactical discussions of medico-political matters (see e.g. *BMJ*, 15 June 1901, p. 1500). The 'infamous conduct' resolution was moved again at the June 1901 meeting but not seconded (*BMJ*, 15 June 1901, p. 1500). Immediately afterwards an attempt was made to increase the representation of GPs, but this also failed. New arguments began to be used, and old ones began to be put in more strident terms. In particular, some doctors argued more vigorously that contract practice inherently led to the neglect of patients (see e.g. *BMJ*, 2 February 1901, p. 288). (This contention that club doctors deliberately provided an inferior service to club patients will be considered in detail below.)

Pressure on the GMC continued and in November 1901, in a major turning point, 'canvassing' was held to be infamous conduct. And a year later came a second equally important decision. The previous year, a resolution declaring advertising to be 'infamous conduct' had not been seconded, but in 1902 the GMC resolved that it was indeed infamous. The case concerned a doctor in Birmingham who had issued handbills in a poor district of Birmingham. One circular had announced that he would provide a free service for the poor, and a second that he would make a token charge of 3d. This was issued because he had been inundated by the response to the first circular. He said in his defence that his aim had been purely charitable. The Medical Defence Union, which had led the case against him, said that the circulars had been issued with one intention only: to take patients from other medical men. The GMC seem to have concurred and told him that they took 'a serious view' of his conduct (*BMJ*, 29 November 1902, pp. 1721–2).

The decisions of 1901 and 1902 were the first occasions on which the powers of the GMC had been openly used to further the pecuniary interests of doctors at the expense of patients. The significance of these decisions was well understood at the time. The decision against canvassing aroused much press interest, and accusations that the GMC had become an instrument of 'trades-unionism' were rife. Hitherto the majority of doctors on the GMC had honourably refused to abuse the power at their disposal. The 1901 decision signalled the arrival of a new majority on the GMC, a majority willing to abuse the power of the state for sectional ends. As E.M. Little, the BMA's historian, was to comment: the profession now found weapons 'placed in its hands which it did not fail to use with effect' (1932, p. 205). Competition, with all its advantages for the consumer, was no longer only something which might upset one's colleagues – it might lead to the loss of a doctor's livelihood. And the BMA were not slow to point this out to recalcitrant colleagues. A series of reports published in the *BMJ* in 1903 reveals that the GMC ruling played a significant part in the battle of the clubs. In that year the *BMJ* published a series of accounts of successful campaigns which had been conducted up and down the country. This included Durham, Gateshead, Walsall, and Rotherham (*BMJ*, 6 June 1903, pp. 1339–41; *BMJ*, 13 June 1903, pp. 1380–81). In these campaigns use was often made of the General Medical Council rulings on canvassing and advertising (see e.g. *BMJ*, 13 June 1903, p. 1381).

And these were indeed two very important weapons. Competition can only work if the flow of information to the consumer is not impeded. Canvassing and advertising are the two chief ways in which information enabling the consumer to differentiate between producers is made available. It is, perhaps, no coincidence that canvassing went first, for the advertiser simply places new information about price or quality before the consumer. The canvasser, by contrast, actively draws the consumer's attention to the merits of the proffered service or product. Both are vital to the protection of the consumer' interests; and both were effectively outlawed by the GMC after 1902.

Capturing the State – the Effects on Professional Power

What difference did the canvassing and advertising rulings make to professional power? In Chapter 2 the evidence revealed that doctors made many attempts to establish local monopolies, but that successes were few and far between. Did the GMC decisions of 1901 and 1902 alter the balance of power?

The pressure on the General Medical Council had been exerted against a background of concerted campaigns all over the country. A highly publicized campaign against the friendly societies was fought by the Southern Ireland branch of the BMA. With full *BMJ* backing, pressure was put on the Cork friendly societies for an increase in fees and the introduction of a sliding scale according to income. The *BMJ* reminded the friendly societies that, at the time, they were 'accustomed . . . to the professional assistance of doctors of good standing' who earned part of their income from patients who paid private fees and part from contract practice. The friendly societies were warned that if more of the doctors who were engaged in contract practice began to be exclusively so engaged, the general standard of care would deteriorate (*BMJ*, 1 December 1894, p. 1254; see also 8 December 1894, pp. 1322–3).

The *BMJ* emphasized that 'we say nothing against the cooperative or provident principle, which, properly worked, is capable of great good, both for the working classes and the doctors.' But 'a one-sided cooperation' was 'capable of great tyranny'. And, contended the *BMJ*, a level of fee had been proposed to the Cork clubs 'below which honest service' could not be rendered (*BMJ*, 15 December 1894, p. 1398; see also *BMJ*, 12 January 1895, p. 103).

By this time the medical journals were boycotting medical

institutes. In 1894 the Leeds FSMA attempted to place advertisements in the *BMJ* and the *Lancet* for an assistant medical
officer. The *BMJ* claimed to be awaiting the outcome of the
GMC's deliberations and the *Lancet* said it did not insert advertisements from medical aid associations (*Oddfellows Magazine*,
March 1894, p. 81). By 1900 warning notices against taking certain lodge appointments were appearing in the *BMJ* and by 1906
warnings concerning twenty-two districts were outstanding
(*BMJ*, 14 April 1906, p. 876).

At the same time the BMA was steadily increasing its recruit-
ment of doctors. In 1895 it still had less than half of registered
doctors. By 1895 there were 33,601 registered medical practitioners, and the BMA had 15,669 members. In 1900 there were
about 36,000 registered doctors, around 50 per cent of whom
were BMA members. The proportion was rising, but only
slowly, in the years leading up to the 1911 National Insurance
Act. In the year before, 1910, there were 40,000 registered doctors, 55 per cent of whom were BMA members.

In 1905 the BMA published a major investigation of contract
practice, carried out by its Medico-Political Committee. The
committee had circularized 12,000 doctors and received replies
from 1,548. Of these, 692 were not engaged in contract practice
and 856 were. Of those who answered the question about pay
rates, 458 replied that their own rates were too low, and 165 that
they were satisfied. Rates of pay among doctors serving friendly
societies or similar clubs varied as follows in the 1,641 cases
reported to the BMA inquiry.

TABLE 1 **Doctors' Pay in Contract Practice, 1905**

Rate of Pay	Proportion of Doctors
2s and under 3s	8%
3s and under 4s	16%
4s and under 5s	53%
5s and over	24%

Thus, about a quarter of clubs were paying less than 4s, and
about three quarters 4s or more. About a quarter paid 5s or
more.

The most common figures were 4s 0d or 4s 4d. This was due to
the convenience of collecting a penny a week. Most large

friendly societies paid the whole 4s 4d direct to the doctor. In the AOF, for instance, the whole of the medical contribution was paid direct to the doctor, with only the 'odd exception' (RCPL, 1909, Appendix VII, Q. 77408). But it was common for some of the smaller societies to pay the doctor 4s 0d, retaining 4d for the cost of administration. This was very cheap compared with doctors' private clubs. Usually doctors paid their collectors from 10 to 25 per cent of the total contributions (BMA, CPR, 1905, pp. 12–13).

Of the 458 who said their rates were too low, 393 suggested the rates that would satisfy them. About 70 per cent of them proposed rates between 4s and 6s per year, and just under half would have been satisfied with 5s or less. These aspirations were gradually being met. And during the early years of the twentieth century doctors' rates of pay were increasing slowly from around 4s to nearer 5s on the average. But the friendly societies were still very reluctant to accept a wage limit prohibiting those earning above a certain income from joining. In the BMA survey there were 542 doctors who declared their support for a wage limit to exclude the well-to-do, and only fifty-five against, although a further seventy-seven regarded it as 'impracticable'. Of those who proposed a wage limit, over 91 per cent would have been satisfied with a £2 per week limit, and over 50 per cent with a 30s a week limit (BMA, CPR, pp. 35–7). Here doctors' aspirations were disappointed. Even where doctors were well organized they continued to be unable to enforce wage limits. In Newcastle upon Tyne, for instance, the Medico-Ethical Society had been strong enough to prevent the extension of club practice to women, but not to impose a wage limit (RCPL, 1909, Appendix Vol. V, appendix CI (25–6, 29)). This was the pattern throughout much of the country. To agree to any such limit seemed to many friendly society members to strike at the whole root of their fraternal philosophy. The Oddfellows, said one leading article in the *Oddfellows Magazine*, prided themselves 'in the entire equality of rank amongst their brethren'. The doctors' wage limit would divide the members into two groups: 'the opulent and the needy'. To be on the doctor's list would be looked upon as 'a mark of social inferiority' (April 1897, p. 101). Such views were widely held. In March 1901 the National Conference of Friendly Societies resolved against accepting a wage limit.

They could not accept such an 'absurd dictum' under any circumstances (*Foresters Miscellany*, April 1901, p. 452).

The friendly societies took particular exception to the opinion sometimes voiced by doctors that contract practice was a charitable service. The view of some doctors is well described in the *BMJ* of March 1895. Contract practice was compared with Poor Law medical attendance. According to the *BMJ*, fees for attendance on paupers were low on two understandings. First, that patients were seen as far as possible at fixed times, and second that home visits were to be kept to a minimum. At that time the *BMJ* felt that between the Poor Law system and open competition for private patients (in which competition fixed prices) there was room for 'an associated system'. But three essential conditions should apply: (a) that patients must accept home attendance as their turn came in the doctor's rounds; (b) that they should come to the surgery at fixed hours and (c) that there should be a wage limit. The only way to offer more reasonably priced medical attendance was to see a large number of patients 'and this can only be done by method and system – things to which the ordinary private patient has a rooted objection'. The private patient wanted to be seen when he liked, and this cost more. The *BMJ* agreed that the avoidance of bad debt was an attraction, but argued that contract practice could still only be worthwhile if it was (a) 'a stepping-stone to something better'; and (b) worked alongside private practice. Without a wage limit there would be no private practice (*BMJ*, 23 March 1895, pp. 657–8).

For the *BMJ* there was a degree of charity involved in contract work:

Between the pauper poor and those people who can afford to pay ordinary fees there are great classes who certainly cannot pay those fees and yet are honest, self-respecting workers. Till the pinch of sickness comes they are independent, and they send for the doctor, in all honesty intending to pay. But, after a long illness, pay they cannot, and without clubs a large proportion of them would fall practically on the charity of the medical profession – an unthanked and unadmitted, but still none the less real, gratuitous medical service. As against this drain on the profession, enforced by that public opinion which does not hesitate to say that a doctor should 'in common humanity' go when sent for, the clubs are at any rate a certain protection. They are better than repudiated or bad debts, and that feeling, no doubt, has influenced many men to accept them at rates which are really unremunerative.

Contract practice had in it 'if properly carried out, an element of charity; it does not pay; the doctor could not live on it alone' (*BMJ*, 23 March 1895, p. 657).

This view was intensely disliked by all working-class institutions. Probably typical of rank and file feeling were the words of one member of the Pendleton Provident Dispensary in Salford. At the annual meeting a doctor commented that the dispensary was intended for those who could not afford to pay medical fees and not for the wealthy. By the 1890s many of the once-charitable provident dispensaries were benefit societies, supported wholly by members' subscriptions. And a member from the body of the hall rejected the doctor's implication that the dispensary was a charity: 'It was a provident and not a charitable or philanthropic institution. It might as well be said that a cooperative society was a charitable institution because its members could not afford to pay the extortionate charges of some shopkeepers' (*BMJ*, 1 February 1896, p. 288). The view that to join a medical club was to 'accept charitable aid' was regularly and vigorously refuted by friendly society members. The medical officer did not mete out charitable aid. He was an honoured equal. As the Chief Registrar of Friendly Societies reported in 1901, the friendly societies desired to pay a fair price for their medical service. They were 'neither beggars nor sweaters'. As one leading article in the *Oddfellows Magazine* saw it, contract practice was simply good business. It was no more than good commercial practice to discount ordinary fees in return for a regular income, freedom from book-keeping, and from the risk of bad debts. The lodge secretary did after all take over some of the administrative functions which would otherwise have had to be performed by the doctor or a paid assistant (*Oddfellows Magazine*, April 1897, p. 99; see also February 1890, p. 48). The doctor's income came regularly, and it was collected either without any charge or for a trifling sum compared with the cost of employing collectors. The doctor also avoided the need to prepare personal accounts, a wearisome task for many.

Moreover, the lodges cooperated with doctors in keeping their costs to a minimum. It was customary, for example, for all medicine bottles to be returned to the doctor. Failure to return a bottle would result in having to pay for it. And the friendly societies tried to encourage members not to make unreasonable demands for home visits.

Very important, too, was the freedom from bad debts which the contract system offered. Without contract practice doctors often found themselves practising for less than club rates. Doctors had learnt from experience that without club practice they faced a 'very large proportion' of bad debts (*Lancet*, 18 February 1871, p. 239). This had long been a problem. In 1846 a census in Scotland showed that 208 out of 253 doctors had not only on occasion treated patients free of charge, but that they had also given them food, wine and clothing. According to one contemporary estimate, one third of the work of Scottish doctors in the 1840s was done for nothing (Turner, 1958, p. 200).

The canvassing and advertising bans seem to have had little impact on the expansion of the medical institutes. They were continuing to prosper. In April 1909 the FSMA alone had thirty-one associations affiliated to it, with a total membership of 283,983. The FSMA was particularly strongly opposed to a wage limit. Doctors reserved their most vigorous measures for the medical institutes but their progress continued. At the Friendly Societies Medical Alliance annual conference in 1911 it was reported that in some areas hospital doctors were declining to accept patients recommended to the hospitals by FSMA doctors. And in a majority of cases consulting surgeons were declining to accept cases referred by medical institute doctors (*BMJ*, 29 April 1911, p. 1013).

In England alone in 1910, the last year before National Insurance, medical institutes reached the peak of their influence. In that year there were eighty-five medical institutes registered as friendly societies, with 329,450 members. Assuming (based on 1896 figures) that unregistered societies comprised around 13 per cent of the total there would have been (as suggested by the only contemporary estimate) about a hundred institutes in 1912, with a membership of approximately 350,000. About thirty of the medical institutes owned their own surgeries and dispensaries (RFS, *Annual Report*, 1918; Comyns Carr, 1912, p. 193; *Foresters Directory*, 1896; Little, 1932, p. 205).

At the turn of the century, notwithstanding the campaigning

of the *BMJ* and *Lancet*, opinion among doctors remained divided. Some were favourable to contract practice; others had their criticisms but saw advantages which outweighed the disadvantages; others, in the view of the *BMJ*, were 'entirely under the thrall of club managers' (*BMJ*, 6 June 1903, p. 1339). That there was no unanimity among doctors was obvious from the comments made by doctors on the 1905 survey forms. Some doctors were bitterly hostile to club practice; others very sympathetic. Those who supported club practice did so for many reasons.

Not least among these reasons was that, notwithstanding the complaints of some doctors, for others it was often lucrative. For the well-established doctor, club practice was a valuable source of income if the practice was otherwise financially viable. Looked upon as a marginal cost, club practice added little to the ordinary overheads of the established doctor and only a little to his drugs bill, and therefore represented a real cash gain (*Lancet*, 14 December 1872, p. 857).

The majority of respondents to the 1905 survey were hostile to contract practice. One London doctor claimed that he lived in physical terror of his club members:

Club members who come to my house are sometimes tipsy and insolent. Sometimes they insult the servant girl and terrify my family. . . Yet I dare not complain. . . My wife and family have been driven out of my own house by drunken members, and forced to seek the protection of neighbours; and because my next door neighbour cleared the noisy club members out somewhat roughly, I was asked to resign by the majority of the club. . . Club patients are far more exacting than private patients, and are seldom friendly in feeling towards the doctor. . . (BMA, CPR, 1905, p. 40).

The critics of contract practice displayed a tendency to express themselves in strident language. Terms like 'slavery' and 'sweating' abounded. But during these years there were other doctors who took a more sober view. One club doctor of twenty-six years' standing challenged the tendency to refer to contract practice as 'slavery'. The doctor had to attend messages from contract and private patients, and this became most onerous when the private patient left town without paying the bill. He conceded that he had sometimes been called upon by hypochondriacal patients, but so had the most fashionable of private prac-

•

titioners. The only difference was that the private practitioner had to 'spend half an hour or more in humouring a good and lucrative patient', whereas the doctor in contract practice could 'in two minutes express his sentiments in good Saxon English'. Consider, he suggested, 'the slavery of the tall hat and brougham'. In contract practice he could dress more comfortably, and avoided the 'fatiguing small talk' which was the lot of many doctors. The private practitioner also had the 'slavery of the day-book ledger' and the task of sending accounts to patients. There was the indignation one felt towards the well-to-do who habitually challenged their accounts, not to mention the annoyance caused by those who refused to pay until forced to do so by legal proceedings. It was impossible to keep bad debts within reasonable limits without employing a collector. He concluded: 'I must confess . . . I should be only too glad if a scheme could be devised by which I could take all my patients on contract' (*BMJ*, 18 February 1911, p. 405).

Some doctors complained that it was necessary to take all the patients of a particular club, whereas in private practice disagreeable persons could be refused. Some found that clubs were dominated by those they regarded as disagreeable. But doctors who complained about the domination of clubs by unreasonable members were told by one London doctor that this was their own fault: 'Once a doctor is known to be one who scrupulously observes his part of the contract he can safely "sit upon" the unreasonable few.' But it was necessary for the doctor to spare the time it took to gain that reputation first (BMA, CPR, 1905, p. 53).

For those doctors who were militantly opposed to contract practice, the results of the 1905 survey must have been a disappointment. The response rate was rather low, about 13 per cent in total. But more important, a surprisingly large number of doctors expressed views favourable to contract practice. Their chief dissatisfaction was over rates of pay, and their demands even in this respect were rather moderate. Given that the enquiry had been set up with the express intent of righting a supposed wrong, it is surprising that a still more unfavourable response was not achieved. Here are some examples of the favourable responses:

Generally speaking, my relations with the club have been of the most pleasant kind. I consider I am quite fairly paid for an average year's work. I have no doubt whatever that if I should request an increase I could get it. I should be inclined to resent any interference by the British Medical Association or any other body between me and my clients (Doctor from North Lancashire town) (BMA, CPR, p. 45).

. . . it is the fairest way for the doctor. . . But the remuneration is too small (Doctor from town in Durham) (ibid., pp. 45–6).

The Friendly Societies, in my opinion, are doing splendid work, and when the medical officer gives reasonable attention to the members, are very desirable appointments. . . They are worthy of all support by the medical profession (ibid., p. 50).

Never had anything but the most cordial relations with any of my clubs (Doctor from South East London) (ibid., p. 41).

In the wake of the contract practice report the BMA asked all its divisions to express a view on the following: 'That it is inevitable in present conditions that there should be in some parts of the United Kingdom some system of contract medical service of the poor.' Sixty-nine replied, only one of which considered contract practice unnecessary. In view of this recognition of the necessity for contract practice the BMA took the view that it should be retained, but that as far as possible it should be organized by doctors and not lay organizations. To this end the establishment of 'public medical services' run by doctors without lay involvement, was encouraged.

As a result of the 1905 inquiry the BMA also considered a set of model rules for public medical services. A set of model rules was published by the Representative Meeting in May 1910. In the intervening years the BMA had been trying to impose new conditions on the friendly societies. Considerable discussion had taken place, but the main sticking point in the discussion between doctors and friendly societies was not the rate of pay, but the wage limit. The doctors had not been able to impose their view.

In February 1909 a meeting between representatives of the friendly societies and the BMA was held under the aegis of the Charity Organization Society. A reasonably friendly exchange of views took place. But no agreement was reached on a wage limit. Friendly societies disliked the idea intensely. At these meetings some doctors demonstrated their fondness for hyperbole. At the February 1909 meeting, Sir Thomas Barlow had said that the life of the club doctor was one of 'absolute slavery'. He would rather cut off his right hand than become a club doctor. A friendly society delegate pointed out that this might be true of some doctors, but he cited the case of another who insisted that £100 of the purchase price of a medical practice should be payable only if the incoming doctor was appointed to the position of local lodge surgeon, as his predecessor had been. Some doctors, he commented wryly, were so opposed to lodge practice they insisted on putting a high price on it (*Oddfellows Magazine*, July 1909, p. 411). Nor was it uncommon for doctors to buy and sell the contract side of a practice along with the private side. As Bro. Barnes, a former grand master of Manchester Unity, told a packed meeting of friendly society delegates in the Albert Hall in 1911, one doctor had lately paid a sum of five times the annual value of his contract practice: 'A very astonishing thing it is', said Bro. Barnes, 'that these doctors are so innocent, so unsuspecting, so unbusinesslike, such children in these things that they pay five years purchase for that which is not worth having.' In fact this doctor was not appointed by the friendly society and so had paid five years' income for the goodwill he did not receive. It was only for this reason that the case came to light (*Foresters Miscellany*, November 1911, p. 742).

There were two further meetings later in 1909, chaired by the former Chief Registrar of Friendly Societies, Sir Edward Brabrook. The doctors sought the replacement of friendly society contract practice by public medical services run entirely by the medical profession. One meeting adopted a resolution approving the desirability of giving members the option of obtaining medical attendance from 'any medical man willing to grant it on club terms', but otherwise no progress was made. Other meetings were also held under Brabrook's chairmanship, but again no progress was made (*Foresters Miscellany*, September 1909, pp. 390–1).

The attitude of friendly society leaders in the years before 1911 was conciliatory. They tended to agree that capitation fees should be higher and encouraged branches to raise pay rates. But the chief reason that they did not rise as far as they might was the sometimes fierce competition between doctors. For instance, J.L. Stead, the Foresters' permanent secretary, told the Royal Commission on the Poor Laws that he personally regretted the low level of fees, but he insisted it was due to competition: 'In my experience in some of the larger towns, I find, I am sorry to say, that medical men are offering privately to do the work at a less figure than the medical men already appointed are doing it at' (RCPL, 1909, Appendix VII, Q. 77528). Thus, on the question of pay the attitude of the friendly societies was conciliatory, although they were implacable on the wage limit issue. This 'class' distinction, they could not accept. The leadership of the BMA did not return the feelings of the friendly society leaders, despite the good feeling between many local doctors and the lodges. From the way the BMA conducted itself during this period, it is difficult to resist the conclusion that they were intent on the destruction of friendly society contract practice. And whilst this remained their long-term aim, they sought in the meantime to impose on the friendly societies new rules more favourable to the doctors. Dealings with local friendly societies were conducted in an imperious manner, and achieved little except to raise hackles. For example, the secretary of one BMA section wrote in these terms to local friendly societies:

I am desired, on behalf of Drs [name], [name] and [name], medical officers to your Friendly Society to inform you that new rules and regulations for the conduct of contract practice, as applied to sick and benefit societies within the area of the section, have been drawn up, and agreed upon by the local section of the British Medical Association. I enclose a copy of these rules and regulations which will come into force on and after January 1st, 1910 and which are binding on all medical men practising within the [named] district. . .

And, societies were told, no medical officer would continue in post after December 1909 unless BMA rates of pay and the new conditions were adopted. The main requirements were: a fee of 1s 0d for every examination; annual rates of 5s for single persons, a family rate of 25s for a man, wife and children under fourteen, or if there were less than five persons, single rates would apply; no attendance or medicine to be supplied for one month after joining; surgery extra; doctors to be on boards of management; and a wage limit of 45s a week (*Foresters Miscellany*, January 1910, pp. 4–7; AOF, *Quarterly Reports*, 1910, pp.

83–4). To lay down the law in this manner was to tell the societies that the rules of their *own* societies were being changed by outsiders. Men who were proud that, despite their humble origins, they had created and sustained fine self-organized institutions, which the great majority of manual workers had joined, did not take kindly to such moves. It made them all the more determined to resist.

Private Practice and Charity

I have focused overwhelmingly on the struggle between the organized consumer and the organized producer as the best test available of the extent of producer power. But some observations should also be made about the charity sector and private practice.

Most free medical care was provided by the outpatient departments of the voluntary hospitals, but also important were the free dispensaries and medical missions. Were any of these institutions run in a manner which offers support for the 'inevitable monopoly' thesis? The free dispensaries and medical missions were run by lay committees and their medical officers were subject to the same sorts of competitive pressures as doctors in contract practice. We do not therefore find in these institutions evidence of a monopolistic medical profession.

Can the same be said of the voluntary hospitals? The top consultants were the dominant power within each hospital. Their reputations had been made in successful private practice, and it was private practice that gave them their continued prosperity. Hand in hand with their success went a duty to care for the poor without charge. This obligation was discharged out of mixed motives. For many there was genuine benevolence. There was also self-interest, in the form of the prestige that went with holding a consultancy in a voluntary hospital, and there was the fact that caring for the poor offered the chance to deal with 'difficult' or 'interesting' cases which might not otherwise be encountered.

This system did not facilitate monopoly. It was based on competition. There was rivalry between consultants and aspiring consultants for private patients, rivalry in which success depended on skill, reputation, and price. There was rivalry between voluntary hospitals, and there was competition between the old-established voluntary infirmaries with their general caseloads and the emerging specialist hospitals: eye infirmaries; ear, nose and throat hospitals; skin disease hospitals; children's hospitals; women's hospitals. And there was rivalry between hospital doctors and general practitioners – rivalry which militated against professional unanimity. The referral system emerged slowly as a partial solution to the resentment of GPs, but it has always been strong, and has continued to some extent to the present day. In addition GPs (and some hospital doctors) complained that too many patients were attended free of charge. Because many could have paid fees, private practice was undermined. This complaint was voiced throughout the life of the voluntary hospitals, although the introduction of hospital almoners to adjust or waive fees according to income went some way towards meeting it.

In the case of private practice it is difficult to make a general judgement about the relative power of the professional and the consumer. In some localities it seems likely that doctors agreed on minimum fees and enforced them. But there was much competition and, until advertising was banned by the GMC in 1902, doctors would often compete by distributing handbills stating their fees. The advertising ban reduced the information available to the consumer. Doctors did charge different fees according to income, and generally adopted the approach of charging what the market would bear. Two pressures militated against this. First, there was competition, and there were always some doctors willing to charge fees below cartel rates. Second, bad debts were a significant problem. Sometimes as much as 40 per cent of a doctors' accounts might be unpaid, although in the case of 'established practices in which the doctor has eliminated those who will not pay', 10 per cent was a more typical level of bad debt (*BMJ* Supplement, 6 July 1912, p. 30).

Supply and demand determined private fees. Medical care was available at different prices designed to suit the ability of consumers to pay. (I will deal with the question of standards in Chapter 4.) Official fee tariffs varied with income (see below p. 90) but actual fees were lower than the official tariff, due to competition.

According to the BMA, the 'recognized standard fee' for home attendance on the 'artisan classes' was 2s 6d, including medicine valued at 5d. But lower fees were 'frequently charged', and anyway charging conventions varied from place to place (*BMJ* Supplement, 6 July 1912, p. 30). Doctors complained about competition for private patients as much as they did about competition for contract patients. One doctor, for instance, told the BMA inquiry: 'Call a monster meeting in London of medical men and let us . . . strike the men off the Medical Register who accept 6d, 1s, or anything less than 2s 6d for advice and medicine' (BMA, CPR, 1905, p. 58).

So, fee levels preferred by the organized profession were still not obtainable on the eve of National Insurance. In some localities it seems likely that there were successful cartels, where atomized individuals faced an organized profession. Ironically those consumers most at the mercy of local professional cartels were the relatively well-to-do. Manual workers had their friendly societies to protect them.

The Marketplace and Monopoly: Conclusions

In the medical marketplace we have found constant efforts being made to establish professional monopolies. In the sense that there were repeated *attempts* to create monopolies we can speak of a tendency to monopoly – the producers were always on the look out for monopoly gains. But this, plainly, is not the same as a tendency for monopolies to emerge successfully. Indeed, if there was a tendency, it was for professional cartels to be inherently unstable.

Monopoly power before the GMC bans: A wide variety of outcomes emerged from the early professional agitation. Supply and demand were the chief determinants of capitation fees. An important factor on the demand side was the inclination of local groups of medical consumers to drive the hardest bargain they could get. Some sought the lowest price; whilst many others struck a bargain which seemed to them to be 'fair' to both sides. In the 1850s and 1860s capitation fees sometimes went very low, occasionally as low as 1s 0d per year. In other cases clubs willingly paid well above the lowest prevailing rates as a mark of the esteem in which their medical officer was held.

What does this tell us about the tendency of free markets to produce monopolies? Certainly we find doctors entering into combinations intended to raise medical fees. And they met with some success. But generally this was the result of mutual agreement. It was not forced on the medical consumer. Whenever professional trade combinations met determined opposition they were defeated. It was almost always possible for medical clubs to bring in other doctors. And frequently they did not have to seek outsiders; outsiders willingly offered themselves. The organized consumer was usually more powerful than the organized producer, and in a few localities at least, a situation, not of monopoly, but of monopsony existed. Doctors could not unilaterally determine fees (though fees were rising by the consent of both parties); they could not impose an income limit to exclude the well-paid; and they could not stop the establishment and growth of medical institutes. They did succeed in inhibiting the extension of most forms of contract practice to women and children, but only at the cost of encouraging the development of medical institutes and the increased use of the free outpatient departments of the voluntary hospitals.

Monopoly power after the GMC bans: As their efforts to establish monopolies failed, we found not only concerted efforts to combine in the marketplace, but also efforts being made to use the power of the state to make financial gains at the expense of consumers. The more extreme demands made by some sections of the profession were not acceded to, but the limitations on advertising and canvassing put considerable limits on competition. This abuse of the powers of the General Medical Council significantly increased the power of the profession at the expense of the consumer. But the organized consumer still retained considerable strength. Even with the additional power given them by the decisions of 1901 and 1902, doctors were still unable to impose desired price increases on consumers; income limits to exclude the higher-paid wage earner from contract practice were few and far between; and medical institutes employing full-time salaried doctors against the wishes of the BMA were expanding rapidly up to 1911.

In the contract practice sector the chief casualties of the canvassing and advertising bans were the medical departments of the commercial insurance companies. The very poor often turned to the insurance companies because they offered medical aid as a loss leader to attract life assurance business. The GMC bans therefore had the unintended effect of reducing provision for the very poor.

The canvassing and advertising bans probably had the greatest impact on private practice. Price competition became far more difficult, and in particular the bans made it far more difficult for young doctors to establish themselves. This may have had a paradoxical effect. Because doctors just embarking on their careers found it more difficult to attract private patients, more of them may have been driven to seek out the alternative of contract practice. This may explain why the canvassing and advertising bans did not significantly alter the power of those medical consumers organized in the friendly societies.

Thus, the evidence so far adduced tends to support the second of the theories of monopoly identified at the outset: professional gains at the expense of the consumer tend to be greater, not in a free market, but when the professionals have at their disposal the coercive power of the state. Until 1911 the chief source of such power available to the profession was the General Medical Council. In Chapter 11 I will consider what difference, if any, was made by the 1911 National Insurance Act, a measure very considerably shaped by professional lobbying during the passage of the bill through parliament.

4

The Consumer's Irremediable Ignorance

The second market failure identified in the Introduction was the 'agency relationship'. Because of the dominant knowledge of the doctor it has been argued that ordinary consumer choice cannot operate. Three main reasons are given.

1. Consumers of most goods and services always have less information than producers about production methods, but, as Professor Kenneth Arrow has argued, the consumer is at least as good a judge as the producer about the utility of a product, and if consumers are initially not well informed they can fairly rapidly learn from experience (1963, pp. 951–2). Medical care is said to be different because, before treatment, consumers have very little idea of the suitability of any particular remedy for their condition. And because medical care is often not repeated, it is more difficult for the patient to learn from experience. It follows that: 'neither before, nor in some cases after, the treatment can the consumer acquire information that will enable him to make an informed choice next time' (Le Grand and Robinson, 1976, p. 38).

This knowledge differential requires the patient to rely on the doctor's judgement, with the result that it is really the doctor, and not the consumer, who shapes any decision about whether or not, and how much, to consume. In such circumstances, some critics argue that 'the market will provide an incentive for exploitation rather than efficiency' (Le Grand and Robinson, 1976, p. 38).

2. In addition, the sick person may well be in the weakest possible position to shop around, although this applies to relatively very few occasions such as emergencies. And even when the individual is too ill to shop around for himself, most people have friends or relatives who can be entrusted with the task.

3. Finally, medical intervention is sometimes irreversible and if mistaken may leave the patient disabled or dead. This applies to many other products too. A faulty car repair may ruin the car for good and result in a fatal accident. A shoddy repair to the roof of a house may lead to a fatal accident, and poor electrical repair work may have equally disastrous results. Health care is unique because the direct object of its attentions is human life, and human life is unique.

These factors have led many analysts to believe that consumer choice cannot operate at all in the sphere of health. Professor Abel-Smith, for example, writes that there are 'few fields of consumer expenditure where the consumer is as ill-equipped to exercise his theoretical sovereignty as in health services' (1976, p. 48). And A.J. Culyer goes further. He believes the marketeer 'betrays a naive faith in the capacity of individuals to resolve their own problems': 'the marketeers' image of a prototypical consumer shopping around for the best quality care at the least price, and getting it, is not a phenomenon that is anywhere actually going to be observed' (1982, pp. 38–9).

The evidence so far adduced in Chapters 2 and 3 raises some questions about the truth of the 'ignorant consumer' thesis. But to test the theory satisfactorily, further issues need to be investigated. In the Introduction I distinguished between two groups of 'market failure' theorists. The first group emphasizes the importance of monopoly and the 'agency relationship'. The second group shows an awareness that consumers were in fact dominant until 1911, but believes this had harmful results for doctor and patient alike and contends that government could do much better. In this chapter I will concentrate on the factual beliefs underlying their paternalism, and specifically the belief that contract practice offered a low standard of service.

The Customer was Always Right – But 'Insisted on Cheap Medicine'

One of the main tactics used by the BMA in their campaign of 1911 was to draw attention to the poor quality of contract medical care as they saw it. They blamed the low quality of medical care on competition and consumer dominance. A number of modern scholars appear to have taken the BMA's propaganda at face value. Even Professor Klein is not immune from this tendency:

Not only were the Friendly Societies and Clubs intent on cutting to the bone the annual fee to the doctor; equally it was to their interest to ensure not so much that patients were cured but that they went on working – since sickness absence payments would mean a further drain on their often inadequate reserve funds.

Klein concludes: 'In the circumstances of working-class general practice at the turn of the century, consumer dominance came to mean professional poverty and poor quality medicine. The customer was always right – but the customer insisted on cheap medicine' (1973, p. 63).

This statement is incorrect. In club practice the lowest fee was not always paid, and as we have seen, there was certainly no tendency to 'cut to the bone'. And the general level of contract fees was steadily rising. Moreover, the lowest-paid doctors were those working as assistants to established practitioners. The appearance of the friendly society medical institutes in the marketplace offered these doctors an opportunity to escape from their penury, for the medical institutes paid salaries well in excess of those that doctors were paying their own junior colleagues. The friendly societies thus raised the income floor for the poorest of the medical practitioners.

But is Klein right about the quality of care provided by contract practice? It is true that club doctors and club patients alike sometimes complained about cheap and ineffective medicines. By 1870, moreover, there was a powerful movement among the friendly societies themselves to improve the quality of medicines provided by replacing the lodge system with the medical institutes. Under the lodge system doctors supplied both attendance and medicine for a fixed annual capitation fee, whereas the medical institutes paid doctors a fixed salary and purchased the drugs direct at wholesale prices, employing their own qualified staff to do the dispensing. They prided themselves on supplying only the best, and on supplying nutritious foods into the bargain. So there is, on the face of it, sufficient reason to suppose that standards were not universally satisfactory to consumers. In this chapter I will review the evidence for and against the view that contract practice was a second-class service. And if there is evidence that it was, I will ask whether or not the low standards were the fault of consumer dominance.

Standards in the Early Years

H.W. Rumsey's account of contract practice, published in 1856, has been influential in creating the impression that friendly society contract practice was second rate. Gosden's history of the friendly societies was, for instance, much affected by Rumsey's version of the facts. He cites Rumsey's assertion that the consciousness on the part of the friendly society members that their medical officers were underpaid 'naturally rendered them suspicious as to the proper fulfilment of the contract' (Gosden, 1961, p. 148, from Rumsey, 1856, p. 159). Rumsey uses two main sources: the evidence of witnesses to the Select Committee on Medical Relief of 1854, and his own evidence to the Select Committee on Medical Poor Relief of 1844.

In 1844 Rumsey was acting on behalf of the 1700-strong Provincial Medical and Surgical Association (later the BMA). He felt that friendly society members were generally not satisfied with their medical officers:

They like to have the power of electing him. They expect him to walk in their annual processions, and they thank him for his services at their club feasts, but individually they often complain that they are not sufficiently supplied with medicines and attendance. *Their dissatisfaction, is I dare say, frequently unfounded and unjust; but the consciousness that their medical contractor is underpaid makes the members naturally suspicious about the due fulfilment of the contract.* The whole custom of contracting for clubs and benefit societies is injurious and degrading to the profession; it encourages a lower order of practitioners, half-educated, ill-conditioned men, who are of no benefit to the community. I am far from saying that such is the general character of surgeons to clubs, but the system introduces such men into the profession and lowers it in public confidence and estimation (SCMPR, 1844, Q. 9086; emphasis added).

It is not possible to establish whether his claim that 'half-educated' practitioners were encouraged by the clubs was true, but if it was true it was made impossible for such men to work for a club two years later in 1858. The Medical Act of that year required that 'no person shall hold any appointment as a physician, surgeon or other medical officer . . . to any friendly or other society for affording mutual relief in sickness, infirmity or old age . . . unless he be registered under this Act' (Section 36).

By the 1870s the view that contract practice only attracted ne'er-do-wells is incompatible with the evidence. Indeed the precise complaint of many doctors was just that 'leading' medical men were having to compete (BMA, CPR, p. 56). Throughout the life of contract practice men of calibre acted as club doctors. In 1871, for example, many club doctors in Hampshire were said to be men of standing in the profession (*Lancet*, 1871, vol. 2, p. 322).

Moreover, Rumsey's own evidence is equivocal on some points. Club practice encouraged low-calibre doctors, he says, but not in general; society members were dissatisfied, but their dissatisfaction was frequently unfounded and unjust. Indeed, it emerged under questioning that he was not sure about members' dissatisfaction. He said he had 'not made it [his] business to inquire', but he knew of some complaints (SCMPR, 1844, Q. 9091). And he compared friendly society medical care favourably with that offered in private doctors' clubs. Standards in the private clubs were lower (ibid., Q. 9089).

The select committee received evidence from other witnesses. But they reported that they had found it difficult to investigate the friendly societies because such inquiry was disliked by both the clubs and their surgeons (SCMPR, 1844, Q. 9077). This may well have been because the cloud of illegality still hung over the societies. It was only ten years earlier, in 1834, that the Tolpuddle Martyrs had been transported for swearing an illegal oath while founding the Friendly Society of Agricultural Labourers. But other witnesses were questioned. And they did not share Rumsey's view. A surgeon in the Newmarket Poor Law union reported that the 5,000-odd members of the Independent Labourer's Medical Club, a club run on provident lines, were 'highly satisfied' (ibid., Q. 5702). And in his view the remuneration was fair, taking into consideration that 'charitable feeling which ought to actuate everyone' (ibid., Q. 5740). In West Ham the doctors had opposed the efforts of the Poor Law union to found medical clubs. But a 'very large' benefit society had found the 'utmost disposition in the medical gentlemen to give their assistance'. And the members of this society were satisfied (ibid., Qs 266, 268, 270). This club had in fact elected the doctors who also served as medical officers to the Poor Law union, in spite of active competition from outsiders (ibid., Q. 273).

Asked if he thought the poor would always be able to choose the best practitioners, the chairman of the West Ham Union replied, not 'always', but 'the poor are pretty discreet in these matters'. This was because 'they generally suppose the gentry choose the best' (ibid., Q. 274). And it was quite common for doctors who spent part of their time serving the rich to serve as club doctors also. Sometimes friendly society members were resentful when such doctors left their contract work to an assistant, but even in such cases the senior partner would handle serious illnesses.

The select committee also heard evidence about Grantham. By 1844 the Independent Labourer's Self-Aiding Medical Club had existed for five years. It was run by the Duke of Rutland who gave evidence to the select committee. The club was also run on provident lines and had fourteen medical officers. The Duke had taken the trouble to call personally at labourers' cottages to discover their satisfaction or otherwise with the club. He concluded: 'I must say that it is my firm belief that the attention which the labourers and their families have received . . . has been far superior to any that they have ever received before' (ibid., Q. 5762). Contributions were 2s a year per adult and 1s for persons under sixteen. The club was said to be 'thriving most uncommonly' (ibid., Qs 5759, 5761). The honorary members contributed according to a scale based on property ownership. The Duke was so pleased that he declared himself willing to contribute five times as much if this proved necessary (ibid., Qs 5770, 5771).

The evidence of witnesses to the select committee of 1854 is more supportive of Rumsey's case. Robert Weale, an assistant commissioner and Poor Law board inspector, compared contract practice unfavourably with the Poor Law medical service. He did not think the Poor Law medical service was capable of being improved, but he said he had seen records of attendance by club doctors and, 'club patients do not get anything approaching the attendance which paupers get' (SCMR, 1854, Qs 360, 376). Mr G. Wallis, the senior physician at the Royal Infirmary in Bristol, told the committee that medical aid in sick clubs was 'so very indifferent that the members come to the public institutions very constantly'. And if an individual was ill for any length of time, medical officers sometimes sent patients to the public institutions for the sake of the free medicine (ibid., Q. 28040).

However, the Reverend Oxenden, a rector in Kent, who ran the Barham Downs Medical Provident Society, took the opposite view. He was asked what the comparative attention paid to paupers and his own club members was and testified that it was, 'very decidedly in favour of the attention on members of [his] society'. He also commented on attendance on friendly society members. This, he said, was 'bad, because the remuneration was too small'. But he did not agree with the earlier witness that the poor were satisfied with the Poor Law medical service. They were 'not at all' satisfied in his judgement, and he testified that they were supplied with inferior medicines (ibid., Qs 1375–6, 1385, 1492–1501).

Medical witnesses who criticized contract practice found it difficult to distinguish between standards and doctors' grievances about low fees. Dr Lord from Hampstead told the commission that benefit clubs and provident dispensaries had been 'very beneficial to the mechanics and labouring classes', but he complained that the system was 'frequently carried out injuriously to the fair interests of the medical profession' (ibid., Q. 3240). Mr J. Ellison, a guardian of the poor in Yorkshire, said he had heard 'many complaints' by club members of 'neglect on the part of their medical men'. He felt that the medical attention was not as efficient as it would be if higher salaries were paid. The remedy was therefore in the hands of the clubs themselves. They could appoint fresh doctors who gave better service, or if they were not available at prevailing prices, they could pay more. Generally, he felt that benefit societies should be encouraged (ibid., Qs 2606–13).

Standards at the Turn of the Century

The four signatories of the Minority Report of the Royal Commission on the Poor Laws found that both friendly society members and doctors had complaints about contract practice. The doctors felt they were badly paid and that some club patients could have afforded ordinary fees. Members of friendly societies were said to complain that they received only perfunctory attendance, that doctors favoured committeemen, and that the doctor sought 'to recoup himself by charging fees for all the other members of the family'. In the view of the Minority Report, these mutual recriminations revealed conditions 'inimical to the cure and prevention of disease'. In medical clubs there was 'no idea of prevention, or even of taking precautions against the communication of disease'. Overworked club doctors had no time to take home conditions into account or to advise on a more sanitary or otherwise healthier lifestyle. There was a tendency to supply only the cheapest medicines. And we find the contempt for the working class which was so characteristic of paternalist reformers. The report quoted a club doctor who had told them that:

> To the poor people who crowd his surgery he must be equally subservient. They must not be allowed to grumble about the club medical man; and to ensure their goodwill it is best to treat them more in accordance with their palates than with their symptoms. To satisfy these patients it is necessary to give them a lot of medicine. It must be a dark medicine with a strong taste, preferably of peppermint (RCPL, MR, 1909, pp. 870–81).

The authors were apparently unaware that this 'evidence' about the taste of medicine had the status of a common joke. It was also told the other way round. Patients, it was said, would drink any amount of medicine, as long as it had an *unpleasant* taste. Nonetheless, their low opinion of the working class led them to recommend strongly against the free choice of a doctor. They wanted doctors to be figures of authority (e.g. p. 874). In the view of the Minority Report, clubs were a failure 'both for the patients and for the medical men' (ibid., p. 871). The report was largely the work of the Webbs. Beatrice Webb was a member of the Royal Commission and the findings and arguments of the Minority Report were reproduced in their book *The State and the Doctor* published in 1910. The book attacks the lack of coordination of the marketplace. And it attacks competition, arguing that it damaged health care standards.

More recent scholars have described working-class medical care in very similar terms. This is how Titmuss describes the situation:

> Under . . . contract systems of medical care, doctors had no security of tenure. They could be dismissed at any time. They were forced to compete and tender for these appointments. There was no free choice in the doctor–patient relationship. As they were always liable to be reported to an 'impertinent' lay committee for inattention they felt

unable to resist demands from patients for medicine. They had no right of appeal under the 'administrative law' of these voluntary associations. As full-time salaried doctors they were often 'unmercifully sweated' by insurance companies at rates of pay which worked out at 3d per consultation; they were under pressure to sign certificates and life assurance forms against their medical judgement, and they were expected to canvass for new patients. . .

According to Titmuss, 'the average doctor, caught in the moral void of club and contract practice', found himself purveying and stimulating the use of secret remedies or proprietary medicines, preparations which promised much but cured little. Titmuss goes on:

Low standards of living, combined with the competitive practices of voluntary associations, philanthropic institutions and commercial insurance companies, led to widespread abuses. The medical journals of the period resound with the cries of doctor against doctor about bribery and corruption, the employment of unqualified assistants, the fee-splitting, the canvassing, the underselling and commission-taking. . . (Titmuss, 1968, pp. 235–7).

Some of Titmuss's exaggerations and unsupported assertions have even been repeated by liberal writers (e.g. Goodman, 1980, p. 10).

Professor Gilbert, an American historian, is even more scathing than Titmuss. He writes that for the thirty-nine million people in Britain with incomes below £160 per year 'there was no "system" of medical care at all'. There were a wide variety of 'overlapping, often competing, invariably uncoordinated' medical institutions (1966, p. 303). Some of these were 'excellent, many were bad, but all were inefficient in promoting the physical welfare of the people they were designed to serve' (ibid., p. 304). There were insufficient voluntary hospitals and the Poor Law infirmaries carried the taint of deterrence. The provident dispensaries, friendly society medical institutes, and the friendly society or private clubs offered a 'particularly pernicious' form of medical care:

Medical competition kept both salaries and capitation fees so low that a doctor in club practice was confronted with the options of depriving himself and his family of a viable income; or in order to increase his income with a capitation fee, of soliciting a larger number of patients than he could conscientiously serve; or in the case of a salary, of neglecting his club patients while searching out private, fee paying patients.

Many doctors, in Gilbert's view, practised under what were 'nearly sweatshop conditions' (1966, p. 149). For writers such as these, competition combined with the conduct of the 'ignorant' working class produced a low standard of health care. Does the evidence support this conclusion?

The most frequently cited source is the Minority Report to the Royal Commission on the Poor Laws. It is rare that the Majority Report is quoted, and rarer still for the evidence presented to the commission to be cited. What did the Majority Report say, and is its conclusion supported by the evidence?

On the issue of the standard of medical care the majority of the Royal Commission on the Poor Laws found:

It is true, no doubt, that sometimes poor people pay absurdly small fees for very indifferent treatment, but the incompetent doctor is the exception and not the rule. In rural districts it is generally the case that both rich and poor are treated by the same doctor, who is also the district medical officer. In the towns, the general practitioner in a working class neighbourhood may be quite as competent, if not so wealthy, as the practitioners at the other end of town (RCPL, 1909, *Report*, p. 259).

The Royal Commission felt that there was some justification for the doctors' complaints about low pay, but they also considered it right to point out that this was due to competition (ibid., p. 259).

Did the evidence they received support the conclusions drawn by the majority of the commissioners? In Nottingham Dr Percival, a surgeon at Nottingham General Hospital and district medical officer, told the Royal Commission that he did not think that medical club care was 'insufficient or unsatisfactory'. This, he felt, was because members 'could change their doctor directly'. He was unaware of any dissatisfaction (RCPL, 1909, Appendix IV, Qs 47993–4).

The almoner of the Westminster Hospital told the Royal

Commission that the poor were able to find good doctors (ibid., Appendix III, Qs 33042–4). And Dr Lauriston Shaw, a physician at Guy's Hospital and member of the BMA medical charities committee, testified that if doctors in working-class areas were less able this was because they were near a hospital and would therefore have less chance of seeing 'difficult' cases. Better doctors tended to practise in areas where they would encounter a high proportion of such interesting cases (ibid., Appendix III, Q. 33308). But either way, the working class had available to them competent hospital doctors or, where these were lacking, competent club doctors.

In Birmingham a district medical officer testified that cheap sixpenny doctors had offered a very poor service, but by 1907 they were dying out. There were not many large friendly societies in Birmingham, but those branches in existence were served by doctors of good repute. Birmingham was well provided with organizations offering free medical care. There were three voluntary hospitals, a medical mission, and a free dispensary (RCPL, 1909, Appendix IV, Qs 43998 (43, 48, 58), 44008). Some witnesses thought that the standard of medical care provided by friendly societies compared favourably with that offered by private doctors' clubs. Such clubs, according to the medical superintendent of the Birmingham medical mission for example, offered less satisfactory care (RCPL, 1909, Appendix IV, Q. 44701).

The Royal Commission received evidence that competent doctors served the poor in rural areas. Just about everyone was a member, for instance, of the Frimley medical aid association, a penny-a-week club which had 'good doctors' (RCPL, Appendix III, Qs 29276–86). The former medical officer of health in Yeovil told the Royal Commission that the 'amount and quality' of medical attendance for the poor was 'sufficient'. And the serving medical officer said that in both the dividing societies and the permanent friendly societies medical attendance was perfectly satisfactory (ibid., Appendix vol. VII, appendix LXI (10), appendix XVIII (4)).

Others testified that club doctors did have a lower reputation than hospital doctors, but that this assessment was often wrong. The medical officer to the Newcastle free dispensary said that many people did prefer the hospital or the dispensary to a club believing ('very often' wrongly, he said) that they got better treatment. Many Newcastle club doctors were 'men of repute' (RCPL, 1909, Appendix V, Qs 51557, 51560).

Some medical officers of health were critical of standards in contract practice. They were also critical of curative medicine generally, preferring a more active role for health visitors who would call at people's houses to seek out ill health and unhygienic conditions. The medical officer of health for Hampstead testified that large numbers of the poor in his district were not in medical clubs. Indeed, those among the poor most in need of medical attendance were least likely to join. And he believed that the conditions under which contract practice was carried on were so unsatisfactory that the interests of the community would not be served by its expansion. It was distasteful to doctors, and the club doctor was 'not infrequently' regarded as an inferior kind of practitioner. He knew of several cases when club patients had experienced serious illness and decided to pay. He believed there could be 'no doubt that club patients do not receive the care and attention that is bestowed on private patients'. The rule in medicine should be 'interrogate all the functions', but in a busy club practice it was impossible to inter-rogate even one function with sufficient care. Neither hospital outpatient departments nor club doctors took sufficient account of home conditions. What was required was an extension of the powers of the sanitary authorities (RCPL, 1909, Appendix vol. IX, appendix XLV (29, 30).

The medical officer of health in Norwich also wanted to see greater use of health visitors, but he did not agree that the stan-dard of health care in contract practice was the problem: 'I am satisfied that the health of the community suffers not so much from insufficiency in amount or quality of the medical assistance at present available for the poor . . . as from the delay which occurs before such assistance becomes available' (RCPL, 1909, Appendix vol. IX, appendix XLVI (33)). The medical officer of health in Brighton, Dr Arthur Newsholme (soon to become principal medical officer of health at the Local Government Board) testified that friendly society medical aid was 'usually somewhat better in quality than that in the poorer forms of pri-vate practice, though the payment made per member is nearly always too little to admit of uniformly good work.' Many of the poor joined 'private adventure medical aid associations' and a still larger number paid 6d or 1s fees to private doctors. These arrangements were 'particularly unsatisfactory', it was only 'seldom' that 'efficient' medical aid was given (RCPL, 1909, Appendix IX, Q. 92534 (4IIiv)).

J.C. McVail, the county medical officer for Stirlingshire and Dunbartonshire, was invited by the Royal Commission to produce a special report. In the event he did not criticize the friendly societies for offering a low standard of medical care as such. He favoured the friendly society method of payment by capitation fee, but felt that friendly society medical officers were 'ill paid'. He also attacked the lack of choice offered to members:

a member of a society wishing to obtain its medical benefits has no choice but to go to the one doctor whom the society employs, even though the member has no faith in his skill and no confidence that such skill as he possesses will be exercised. And, on the other hand two or three such members will harass the doctor far more than a hundred others (RCPL, 1909, Appendix XIV, p. 158).

But his evidence seems to have been second hand, because a little later he comments that many friendly societies were financially unsound and that the discontinuance of the payment of doctors' salaries might help them become more sound (ibid., p. 160). No one who had the slightest acquaintance with the friendly societies would have made such a remark. Those societies in financial difficulties faced the problem that their sick funds could not meet their future (and sometimes present) obligations to pay sickness benefit. Doctors' capitation fees were not paid into sick funds, and doctors' salaries not paid from sick funds. Medical care was financed separately, and in most cases the friendly societies acted in effect as collecting agencies, handing over the whole of each member's subscription to the doctors at quarterly intervals. Ending this process would have made no difference whatsoever to any friendly society's financial soundness.

But not all government medical officers were critical of contract practice. The chief medical officer to the Board of Education who had formerly served as medical officer of health in Finsbury, told the royal commission that the friendly societies and provident dispensaries were doing 'a very large amount of good in the prevention of disease and in the cure of disease'. He was, however, very critical of 'cheap doctors' who charged 6d or 1s fees. They did not, in his view, even attempt curative medicine (RCPL, 1909, Appendix IX, Qs 94550, 94594).

Much has been made of the resentment felt by doctors at being sweated. But such feelings were not universal. A district medical officer in Oxford, for example, told the Royal Commission that he found both Poor Law and club work 'remunerative' and that club members were 'very considerate' (ibid., Appendix III, Qs 34125, 34129–30).

Even when doctors did feel resentful, competition meant they could not allow their feelings to affect the way they treated club members. One doctor in Merthyr who earned 12s for families and 6s for single adults (when the average was 8s and 4s respectively) said: 'I rather resent persons coming to me who ought to pay a great deal more; but I do not know that I can afford to show that resentment at all' (RCPL, 1909, Appendix V, Q. 48976). In Suffolk the medical officer of health for Bury St Edmunds was asked if he thought contract patients were neglected. He also replied that competition made neglect difficult: 'You see competition is pretty keen among doctors, and a man soon gets a name for neglecting his club patients if he does it; and the consequence is that somebody else gets them. I do not think there is any neglect' (RCPL, 1909, Appendix VII, Q. 75657).

Among friendly society members there was satisfaction with contract practice in many areas. One Manchester Unity member, also a member of the Cardiff board of guardians, doubted whether the friendly society system could be improved upon (RCPL, 1909, Appendix vol. V, appendix XXVIII(7)). The treasurer of the Swansea Juvenile District of the Rechabites said he 'hardly ever' received complaints about insufficient medical attendance. Perhaps once in every three to four years there were some complaints, 'but as a rule the doctors give every satisfaction to the societies' (ibid., Appendix V, Q. 50843).

The above review of the evidence presented to the Royal Commission does, I believe, fairly represent the views expressed. It seems to me to justify fully the qualified judgement made by the Majority Report. The less balanced view of the Minority Report was the result of neglecting all the contrary evidence.

There was also ample contrary evidence in the BMA's 1905 inquiry report, a source also used by the Webbs.

Moreover, we now know that Beatrice Webb deliberately attempted to manipulate the evidence: 'I do not altogether despair of getting my transference of Poor Law medical relief to the public health authorities accepted by the majority', she wrote, 'I am more or less engineering the evidence in my direction. . .' (1975, p. 370). She also records how she practised 'tacit deception' of fellow members of the Royal Commission. She had been asked by one colleague to let the whole Commission see her correspondence with medical officers of health, on which the Webbs' own report had been based. To prevent them from appraising the whole of the evidence Mrs Webb sent the commissioners only a selection, deliberately biased in her favour. She writes: 'To be frank, I had qualms of conscience in making any kind of selection of those I did and did not send.' But she justified this to herself by taking the view that the commissioner who had requested the information was herself biased: 'So I swallowed the tacit deception and sent exactly what I thought fit – without, be it added, in any way giving the Commission to understand that I had sent them the whole or the part' (1975, pp. 392–3). In short, it can reasonably be inferred that Mrs Webb's own view was biased. A few pages later she writes: 'Fortunately, we have already discovered our principles of 1907, and we have already devised our scheme for reform. What we are now manufacturing is the heavy artillery of fact that is to drive both principles and scheme home' (ibid., p. 399).

Contract practice also had its defenders within the medical profession, even at the height of the conflict over the legislation of 1911. For example, early in 1911 one correspondent to the *BMJ*, a doctor from North Shields, mounted a spirited defence of contract practice. He pointed out that he defended the principle only, not prevailing rates of pay. He had been engaged in contract practice for twenty-six years, alongside ordinary practice. He repudiated as ridiculous the claims of another doctor that 1,500 patients would require fifty visits a day. From his own experience he found that about 1,000 patients worked out at about ten visits a day. He dealt specifically with the accusation that club doctors 'scamped' their work and contended that the reverse was often the case:

So far from the work being scamped, a contract patient often gets more attention than those who have to pay for every visit, and who in consequence try to keep down the doctor's bill by discouraging visits and neglecting medicine, and failing to send when necessary or sufficiently early.

But apart from this, he pointed out that a contract doctor would be a fool not to try to cure his patients quickly, for he would only increase his own work. Moreover:

In an urgent or interesting case one can visit a club patient as often as necessary without incurring the suspicion of mercenary motives, and, on the other hand, one does not have the tiresome routine of visiting a chronic case every day and spending a weary half-hour trying to think of something fresh that will interest a wealthy and exacting patient. My experience is that my contract patients look upon me as a friend, and are pleased to see me not only when they are very ill, but also at any time when I think it necessary to call (*BMJ*, 18 February 1911, p. 405).

Such views were by no means unique among doctors. Nor were they new. In the 1890s doctors challenged the view expressed in the *BMJ* that 'very few club doctors look after their patients properly'. One doctor wrote in to point out that some might, but in his experience, most medical men treated their club patients well. He cited an example of one of his own patients who had suffered from 'bronchopneumonia'. He had visited him on twenty-two occasions, including seventeen consecutive daily visits (*BMJ*, 14 March 1896, p. 672).

The argument that the pay was insufficient to attend club patients honestly and honourably was also refuted by a doctor who was grand master of the Mitcham District of Manchester Unity. He kept records for three years and concluded that at a penny a week he 'could do for them what he could' running accounts for private patients. He emphasized the value of freedom from bad debts. He had written off £40 in the previous three years from people who could have been paying club contributions (*Oddfellows Magazine*, August 1909, pp. 488–9). The *BMJ* had refused to publish his letter and so he had sent it to the *Oddfellows Magazine*.

Contract practice, according to some doctors – and quite contrary to the claim of the Webbs – encouraged preventive medicine. According to an experienced doctor, colliery practice in Durham encouraged a preventive approach. The doctor's work was lessened 'by being called promptly in times of sickness, and by every effort he makes to prevent disease among his clientele, or to instruct them how to deal with the many minor complaints which form the bulk of his daily work' (BMA, CPR, 1905, p. 44).

The claim that private patients were given preferential treatment was explicitly rejected by some medical men. A Kent doctor said: 'The majority of my members are *bona fide* working men, and when they are ill I treat them as private patients and get them well as soon as possible, and it pays me well' (BMA, CPR, 1905, p. 44).

Some doctors, however, do appear to have acted resentfully towards club patients. As one doctor put it, some doctors reasoned to themselves 'well, the club pays us 3s 0d each for medical treatment and medicines. We shall give them just 3s 0d worth' (*Oddfellows Magazine*, December 1889, p. 374). Another doctor suggested that, whilst there might be resentment, this affected the doctor's demeanour, rather than the treatment he offered:

I am ashamed to say that it is impossible to deny the fact that distinctions have been, and are, made in the treatment of contract and private patients by some practitioners. It cannot be denied. I will not say that the distinction exists in the essentials of diagnosis or treatment so much as in demeanour; but the contract patient is often conscious of it, and feels it, and makes it a standing grievance (*BMJ*, 2 December 1905, p. 306).

But club members sometimes suspected that inferior medicines were supplied. Some club surgeons were said to supply either a white or red bottle of medicine. A 'tablespoonful of something' was put in and the bottle filled from the tap (*Oddfellows Magazine*, December 1889, p. 372). And according to the Friendly Societies Medical Alliance (the national association for medical institutes), club patients were sometimes attended by an assistant doctor and thus given second place to private patients. They were treated with 'undeserved harshness' as if they were the recipients of charity. But there were 'many honourable exceptions'. Medicine, felt the FSMA, was also sometimes of an inferior quality and sometimes supplied in inadequate quantities (GMC, 1893, pp. 30–31).

However, the view that it was common to provide club patients with inferior medicines was refuted by a past provincial grand master in Manchester Unity's Sunderland District. In that area there were 'good doctors as a rule for both medicine and attendance'. In his view they were as good as any private patient might desire (*Oddfellows Magazine*, February 1890, pp. 48–9). A former noble grand of a miners' lodge in Derbyshire also refuted the view that 'cheap and nasty' medicine was prescribed. Doctors in that area took it as an honour to be connected with friendly societies, and many were members (*Oddfellows Magazine*, March 1890, p. 82). And a Manchester Unity member told readers of the society magazine about a Norwich doctor who had called on one seriously ill member of Manchester Unity as often as three times a day, Sundays included, during 'many weeks'. This was not a solitary case and the club member believed 'there *never were* and *never will be* many exceptions all the time that the present high moral tone of the medical profession exists' (*Oddfellows Magazine*, August 1889, p. 245).

There were disadvantages of club practice for both doctor and patient. Wealthier potential patients might take the view that a doctor who 'took clubs' only did so because he had failed to command the confidence of sufficient private patients (*Lancet*, 18 February 1871, p. 239). And in some localities fee-paying patients seem to have preferred not to be confused with club patients. Some doctors tried to keep separate waiting rooms to avoid the problem (*Lancet*, 28 September 1895, p. 815). Doctors might, therefore, find themselves looked down upon if their clientele was mixed. But for the very many doctors practising exclusively in working-class areas this made little difference.

The chief disadvantage for the club patient was that sometimes 'paying patients' were seen ahead of them in the queue. But this was not necessarily resented, for often all that the fee was buying was convenience, a fact well understood by all parties. Indeed, from time to time club patients took advantage of this facility themselves. The BMA estimated in 1912 that as many as 20 per cent of friendly society members might prefer to consult a doctor privately rather than use the society medical officer (*BMJ* Supplement, 6 July 1912, p. 30).

The BMA study of 1905 does provide some evidence that consultation rates varied with the capitation fee. The report thought that attendances were, if anything, underestimated (BMA, CPR, 1905, p. 14).

TABLE 2 **Capitation Fees and Average GP Attendances**

Annual Capitation Fee	Members	Average Attendances per annum	Average Fee per attendance (pence)
2s to 2s 11d	9,630	3.59	7.95
3s to 3s 11d	9,311	3.67	10.55
4s to 4s 11d	17,741	4.46	10.98
5s and over	4,211	5.43	13.36
	40,893	4.10	10.60

SOURCE: BMA, CPR, 1905, p. 35.

The average number of attendances was lower for those paying the lower fees. This may have been because patients adjusted their demands, but it is more likely to have been because doctors initiated less consultations. We know from recent studies that many consultations are initiated by the doctor. Cartwright found that, according to patients, about two fifths of visits to the doctor were made on the doctor's initiative (Cartwright, 1967, p. 31).

In 1912 the BMA again investigated attendance rates. They compared rates in private doctors' clubs, provident dispensaries, and friendly society medical institutes. Private clubs averaged 3.75 attendances per member per year, provident dispensaries 6.2, and friendly society medical institutes 5.69. The grand average was 5.5 (*BMJ* Supplement, 6 July 1912, p. 30; also 25 May 1912, pp. 570–1). The private clubs, where the doctor's control was greatest, show lower attendance rates compared with provident and friendly society schemes. Private club fees, however, tended to be higher than friendly society capitation fees. And contributions to provident dispensaries tended to be lower than friendly society rates. So low fees did not automatically produce lower attendance rates, but the 1905 figures do suggest some sort of link.

How do the 1905 rates compare with the findings of more recent studies? A study carried out jointly by the College of

General Practitioners and the General Register Office in 1955–6 found average consultation rates varying from 2.7 to 9.2, with an overall average of 3.8. Other surveys have found rates varying from 3.0 to 5.1 (Cartwright, 1967, pp. 24–5). So even the low rate of 3.59 attendances per annum is not markedly different from rates prevailing in some localities under the NHS.

In some areas, friendly society members themselves complained about standards. Evidence given to the BMA inquiry of 1905 suggests that in the 1880s some club patients in London were dissatisfied with second-class treatment and set up medical institutes as a result (*BMJ*, 22 July 1905, Supplement, p. 53). A former noble grand from Woolwich claimed that 'club patients are invariably subordinated to the private patients, both as to attendance, civility, and medicines, and are often subjected to such indignities as to place them in a position but very little removed from that of paupers' (*Oddfellows Magazine*, January 1893, p. 13). And medical institutes elsewhere were sometimes founded because of dissatisfaction with the standard of contract practice care (*Lancet*, 28 April 1900, p. 1255) and sometimes because of the unreasonable fees charged by doctors in some localities (*Lancet*, 28 December 1895, p. 1647). The FSMA in Chester was established largely as a result of dissatisfaction with the standards prevailing in contract practice (*Lancet*, 28 April 1900, p. 1255; see also *BMJ*, 30 November 1867, p. 513).

Standards did vary. According to the *Lancet*, if a well qualified medical man took clubs he often left this side of the practice to his assistant (*Lancet*, 3 November 1877, p. 654; see also *Lancet*, 3 October 1885, p. 651). Where this happened the friendly societies' response was often to establish a medical institute. At Lincoln the medical institute was established chiefly because the friendly societies were dissatisfied with the standard of medical care being offered by contract practice doctors, and particularly with their use of assistants (*Lancet*, 26 October 1895, pp. 1070–1).

But the establishment of a medical institute can not automatically be taken as evidence of dissatisfaction with club doctors. In Oswestry, Manchester Unity lodges established a medical aid association, chiefly in order to secure attendance for their families. They employed the existing lodge doctor, with whom they were satisfied, at 8s per annum for the member and his family. Confinements cost 10s 6d. The past provincial grand master felt they got the 'best possible attendance' from their medical officer (*Oddfellows Magazine*, June 1890, p. 186).

Standards and Competition: Some Conclusions
The evidence on which I have had to rely has chiefly been the testimony of contemporary participant observers. Each played an active role in the supply or consumption of medical care and each had a self-interest which must be taken into account in weighing the evidence. Many doctors very clearly wanted more pay, and this affected their judgement. They had two particular incentives for exaggerating the extent of second-class treatment. Firstly it was central to their case before the General Medical Council in the 1890s; and secondly, it formed part of their strategy of persuading friendly society members that it was to their advantage to pay higher capitation fees (e.g. Dr Belcher's contribution to the *Oddfellows Magazine*, June 1889, pp. 175–8). The evidence of the friendly society medical institutes was similarly affected. The medical institutes were in competition with lodge practice and, in their efforts to wean members away from the lodge doctor to the local medical institute, they made great play on the superior medicines offered by medical institutes. Defenders of lodge practice may also have had an interest in presenting themselves in a good light.

Leaving such considerations aside for the moment, what picture emerges if the testimony of the various observers is taken at face value? Comment ranges from total condemnation, through qualified criticism, to wholehearted approval. This in itself is of interest, for the leading historians of the period (Titmuss, Gilbert, and Klein) show little or no awareness of the evidence that contract practice offered a satisfactory standard of medical care. Their accounts rely almost entirely on the one-sided criticisms of the medical profession. This alone is sufficient reason to question their conclusions. Moreover, even when professional evidence may have been contradictory, this has not been detected. For instance, doctors repeatedly complained that well-paid people who could have afforded private fees joined friendly societies and took advantage of the services of the lodge doctor. If standards were universally bad, why did people who could afford to pay private fees continue to obtain medical care through contract practice? Unless these well-to-do individuals were complete fools, it seems possible that they may have seen little point in paying large private fees when they could get the same or a similar service for a much smaller outlay.

There is another problem with the way in which the period has been investigated and reported. Academic observers have been both paternalistic and statist in their personal preferences. They have taken the view that (a) the great mass of the people needed to be protected from themselves; and (b) that the answer to any problem is to contemplate what kind of government programme should be introduced to solve it. Voluntaristic solutions have simply not been on their agenda.

As a result of these personal preferences they have placed little value on the judgements of consumers. If a local friendly society branch, say, kept the same medical officer for twenty years (as quite a few did) in spite of the fact that other doctors were coming along and offering to serve the branch for a lower fee, this did not count as evidence that the service was satisfactory. Even if the particular doctor was satisfactory *to the branch members*, as he must have been after twenty years, the branch members were deemed unfit to judge. But in the real world there is no better criterion than the well-informed assessment of the self-directing consumer. (I will deal with the problem of information flow in the next chapter.)

The only reason for ignoring the consumer's judgement is if it can be shown to be ill-informed in the particular case, and that some other person's judgement is better informed in the given case. There is no shortage of 'experts' making a *general* claim that their judgement is always superior to the consumer's. But what credence should we give to their claims?

The contention that their judgements are necessarily superior is based on two common sense observations (that just about everyone would share): (a) that we all make mistakes from time to time, even when our vital interests are at stake; and (b) that when any one of us makes a special effort to study a subject it does not take long to advance beyond the level of knowledge of people who have not made a similar effort. From this common-sense foundation it is tacitly inferred that 'expert' judgements are *always* superior to those of the non-expert. Logically this is nonsense. Moreover, it is a point of view which leaves out of account the fact that the 'expert' may have a self-interest which has costs for the consumer.

However, it is theoretically possible that a consumer might be in a position in which information about producers was too thin to make a well-informed judgement, and in which no mechanisms were available to give effect to such judgements as the consumer *could* make on the performance of producers. From the evidence, was this the situation of the consumer of contract medical care? Was there a flow of information to consumers, and were there mechanisms for taking appropriate action? It seems to me to be quite clear, even from the evidence so far presented, that there were such mechanisms (and I will show below that there was a considerable information flow to the consumer). Each friendly society had a complaints procedure which provided for complaints to be made, heard, and judged. Unsatisfactory doctors were fined for minor breaches, or dismissed and replaced for more serious neglect of patients.

Some doctors felt that the capitation fees were too low to cover the cost of medicines which ought to be prescribed. Other doctors took the view that fees were adequate. Some doctors were said to cut their drug bills by dispensing smaller quantities than they habitually dispensed for private patients, who paid the full cost themselves. For instance, they supplied medicine to last two or three days instead of a week. If this was not enough the contract patient had to return to the doctor for more. This was not clinically harmful to the patient, but was less convenient. More importantly it reflects the fact that in contract practice the doctor bore the cost of drugs, whereas the private patient paid for his own. When paying themselves doctors were more cost conscious. But all cost consciousness is not negligence. What evidence of negligence was there?

Some doctors did dispense 'stock' mixtures and refrained from dispensing more costly drugs. Others, rather than mislead a patient, prescribed an expensive drug but declined to dispense it, advising the patient to pay the extra at a chemist's shop. Still other doctors carried out their duties faithfully, prescribing and supplying drugs they judged to be clinically the most effective. There is evidence that doctors tailored the number of consultations to the fee, but average consultation rates for low payers are not low enough to suggest that doctors seriously neglected patients.

In the case of capitation fees being fixed at a level which made it impossible for doctors to cover the cost of medicines, there were four main mechanisms enabling consumers to remedy the situation. They could take disciplinary action against a poor performer, as their rule books provided; they could replace an unsatisfactory doctor; they could raise the doctor's pay; or they could abandon the flat-rate system altogether by founding or joining a medical institute.

This last strategy was one of 'backward' integration, extending the role of consumer organizations in the delivery of health care. In response to criticisms of club doctors who were felt to devote disproportionate attention to private patients, the medical institutes hired full-time doctors for a salary and forbade them from taking private patients. And in response to fears that some club doctors did not supply the very best of medicines, the medical institutes took over from the doctors direct responsibility for the dispensing of drugs. Of course, *any* cost was not acceptable to consumers. One of the chief reasons for the flat-rate system was precisely to contain the cost of medicines. The friendly societies had experimented with alternative schemes and generally abandoned them as too costly. The problem of cost containment remains with us today, and so it can not be said that a state takeover overcomes it. If a flat-rate system is adopted to put a ceiling on drug costs there will always be a problem of finding the optimum limit. Constant adjustment in the market is a more flexible instrument than a state-imposed limit.

I will describe the disciplinary procedure, to which friendly societies occasionally had recourse, in detail in Chapter 7. In addition to providing a complaints procedure the rules naturally laid down the medical officer's duties. Usually the medical officer was expected to offer all medical care short of hospital treatment. But by the turn of the century changes in medical practice were tending to make this a rather outdated concept. The use of surgery and anaesthetics was becoming more common and more costly. Many rulebooks, for example, required doctors to provide minor surgery without additional charge (BMA, CPR, 1905, pp. 23–24). Such rules were becoming unrealistic, and slowly rulebooks were being changed to permit small extra charges to be made.

I am not here entering into the rights and wrongs of the requirement that minor surgery was covered by the annual capitation fee, nor considering whether rulebooks were changed too slowly or too rapidly; the matter is being investigated purely to establish whether or not the range of services being delivered in return for the capitation fee was controlled by friendly society rules, or by the autonomous decisions of medical men. It is clear that many medical officers felt that to keep their jobs they had to provide services such as minor surgery. They wanted to charge more for such 'extras', but generally they were not able to do so without the consent of the friendly society that employed them. The contention that consumer sovereignty meant cheap and nasty medicine is therefore further refuted. Consumer sovereignty kept down prices, and in some cases doctors were consequently tempted to offer an inferior service, but competition and friendly society disciplinary procedures militated against this deterioration. The rulebooks also served to ensure that doctors offered a wide range of services extending beyond simple advice and medicine, extending to setting fractures, suturing wounds, and minor surgery. As I will show later (pp. 140-41), the 1911 Act reduced the range of these services.

In the medical institutes control was still wider than in club practice, for the patients themselves owned, or at least rented and controlled, the very facilities used by the doctor. Surgeries were kept up to the standards that suited patients; the dispensary was on the same site; a nurse might be available, and so on. One medical institute even required its medical officer (in practice it would have been a servant's task) to ensure that the waiting-room fires were lit by 8 a.m. in the winter (BMA, CPR, 1905, p. 18).

The chief difference between contract practice and private practice was that a private fee bought convenience. Paying, say, 2s 6d for a consultation meant the doctor would arrange an appointment to suit the patient. For 3s 6d, a home visit could be arranged at an agreed time, and not when your turn came in the doctor's rounds. Just as today patients go private to avoid long NHS queues, so before the 1911 scheme they paid fees to avoid having to wait around for the doctor. Occasionally doctors kept

two waiting rooms, one for fee-paying patients and one for contract patients; and sometimes a private patient might be seen in
the private part of the doctor's house and not in the surgery.
From such evidence as there is, this does not seem to have been
the norm, but it was not uncommon. Sometimes these distinctions were the result of, or gave rise to, snobbery. And for many
friendly society members such distinctions certainly rankled
strongly. But the important question is whether a private fee
purchased a more attentive diagnosis and more conscientious
treatment. No doubt there were exceptions, but I can find little
evidence to suggest this was the case. Diagnosis and treatment
do not seem to have differed significantly. Indeed contract practice encouraged doctors to practise preventive medicine rather
than to wait for patients to call. In this sense, and where doctors
accepted the challenge, contract practice was superior to private
practice.

To sum up: can it be validly said that it was competition that
made contract practice an inferior service compared with private practice? The evidence is that low private fees of 6d did go
hand-in-hand with low-quality doctoring. But this was private
practice and not contract practice. Contract practice varied. But
if standards fell below those desired by consumers, it was not
competition that brought this about. On the contrary, it was
competition that gave the consumer the power to improve the
service. In those localities where friendly societies were dissatisfied with the service on offer they could and did discipline their
doctors; they could and did raise fees when appropriate; they
could and did sack and replace their medical officers; and they
could and did found medical institutes to employ full-time doctors and dispense drugs direct. The best protection for the
patient against inferior service by some doctors was the potential service of all other doctors.

5
Were Any Groups Neglected?

The Market and Poverty
A market is said to distribute the best health care to the rich at the expense of the poor. For example, Le Grand and Robinson argue:

If the market system were used to allocate health care, the best health treatment would go to those who could afford to pay the most and thus to those with higher incomes. Poor people might be unable to afford to pay doctor or hospital bills, and would not receive the health care they needed (1976, p. 40).

Were the poor neglected in the pre-1911 market place? The very poorest were treated under the Poor Laws and so my present concern is with the provision made in the marketplace for that part of the population in receipt of low incomes, but not relying on the Poor Laws.

The various kinds of medical club were found by the fourteen-strong majority of the Royal Commission on the Poor Laws to be 'almost universal and within the reach of almost everyone' (RCPL, 1909, pp. 257–8). They also found that there were 'many', including among the 'poorest working class' who preferred to pay as private patients (ibid., p. 259). The Royal Commission had been told by the medical officer of health in Manchester that a 'very considerable' number of persons earning less than 30s a week paid ordinary fees (ibid., Appendix IV, Q. 38390). And there is evidence that this had been so for many years. According to the *Association Medical Journal*, in 1853 'many' workers receiving only 12s to 15s a week paid the customary private fee (22 July 1853, p. 652). This is not as surprising as it may seem, for doctors charged fees according to income, and the lowest level of fee was within the grasp of the low-paid worker. Rent was usually taken as a rough indicator of income. An official tariff in *Whitaker's Almanack* distinguished three scales: those paying rents from £10 to £25 a year; those paying £25 to £50; and those paying £50 to £100 plus. The minimum fee for a surgery consultation for the poorest class was 2s 6d (*Whitaker's Almanack*, 1900, p. 411; McConaghey, 1966, p. 155; Peterson, 1978, pp. 211–13). In fact fees actually charged were much lower. In 1889 the fee for a surgery consultation varied from 1s 0d to 2s 6d. And for a home visit (including medicine) fees varied from 1s 6d to 3s 6d. The most common fees were 2s 0d or 2s 6d, with 1s 6d charged for the very poor (*Oddfellows Magazine*, June 1889, p. 177).

Alfred Cox reports that when he embarked on his career, 1s 0d and 1s 6d were the going rates for surgery consultations and home visits respectively (Cox, 1950, p. 22). On the eve of National Insurance fees had not changed much. In working-class areas it was 'difficult' to charge even 1s 0d per consultation, and among the 'better classes' difficult to charge as much as 3s 6d (*Oddfellows Magazine*, August 1909, p. 489).

Such fees, as long as they had to be paid only occasionally, were within the means of wage earners. In 1906 the average wage of unskilled workers was about 22s a week; for the semi-skilled, about 28s; and for the skilled worker, around 37s a week (Routh, 1980, pp. 100, 106, 113). In addition, in some large manufacturing towns arrangements were sometimes made to pay fees by instalments (BMA, CPR, 1905, p. 9).

The alternatives to fee paying fell into four main categories: charities offering a free service; semi-charities, which covered their costs partly from patient contributions and partly by charitable donations and subscriptions; the insurance companies, which offered medical care as an inducement to buy life assurance; and the self-supporting, self-organizing friendly societies and works clubs. The government's survey of 1910 suggests that many would also have turned to unqualified medical practitioners. In eighty-two out of 217 towns studied, unqualified medical practice was either increasing or taking place in large amount, and in a further seventy-five it existed to some extent. In twenty-seven there was very little, and in thirty none. This included chemists who prescribed over the counter, herbalists, and bonesetters, Christian scientists, faith healers, abortionists, and VD specialists. In mining areas such as Northumberland, Durham and Wales bonesetters enjoyed equal standing with doctors (PMSUP, 1910, pp. 3–4, 8).

Many poor people sought care from the voluntary hospitals and charitable dispensaries, which provided advice and medicine free to those on low incomes. These were available in most large towns. The system at the Newcastle free dispensary was that patients with a subscriber's letter of recommendation received attendance and medicine free, whilst 'casuals' paid 2d for any medicine prescribed (RCPL, 1909, Appendix V, Q. 50566).

Of greatest importance for the supply of free medical care were the outpatient departments of the voluntary hospitals. *Burdett's Hospitals and Charities* (1907) estimated that one in four of the population of London obtained free medical relief in 1877, one in two and a half in 1894, and one in 2.1 in 1904. In 1887, for example, when the population of London was just over four million, there were one and a half million outpatient attendances at London hospitals. In the same year there were also 162,000 consultations at twenty-six free dispensaries; 102,000 at part-pay dispensaries; and 126,000 at provident dispensaries run on benefit society principles for the whole family (*Hansard*, 1889, vol. 338, cols. 1552–5; Abel-Smith, 1964, p. 153). Using figures published by the Hospital Sunday Fund, Arthur Newsholme (later Sir Arthur) estimated the proportion of the metropolitan population obtaining free medical care in 1907 at one in four (*BMJ*, 14 September 1907, p. 658; *Lancet*, 1 June 1907, pp. 1543–50).

Outpatient departments were important in the great majority of large towns, but the London figures are not typical of the country as a whole owing to the heavy concentration of hospitals in the capital. Provincial figures varied. In Newcastle in 1894 the figure was one in 1.8, in Edinburgh one in 2.7, in Glasgow one in 4.9, in Cardiff one in 7.3, and in Portsmouth one in 14.3 (*BMJ*, 14 September 1907, p. 658). In Leicester in 1907, for instance, when the population was around 125,000, the General Infirmary attended 39,994 outpatients and 13,836 casualties, and admitted 2,950 inpatients.

The second alternative to private fee paying was the provident dispensary. These had developed from the free dispensaries, most of which had emerged in the eighteenth century. It was felt that the beneficiaries would feel greater self respect if they were able to pay at least something towards their own health care. They therefore paid a low annual contribution felt to be within the means of the very poor, and the balance was supplied by the honorary members (who did not benefit from the dispensary). The BMA acknowledged that many of those in provident dispensaries, private clubs, public medical services, and medical societies were 'so poor' that they were unable to pay premiums equivalent to the amount that would be paid in a year if they paid fees at working-class rates. In rural districts, in particular, clubs were said to provide for the 'thrifty but very poor' (BMA, CPR, 1905, p. 9). One of the strongest provident dispensaries was the Leicester Provident Dispensary. It had 50,798 members in 1907 and ran a small maternity home and cottage hospital. Fees were a penny a week for adults, half for children; or threepence halfpenny a week for a man, wife and all children under fourteen. The People's Dispensary, also run on provident lines, had 9,000 members (RCPL, 1909, Appendix IV, Q. 47501).

The insurance companies provided a third alternative to private fee paying. They also catered for the poor. Most of their customers had to pass a medical examination. But there was provision for those persons contributing for a very small sum assured to be admitted without a medical examination at the discretion of the agent. The agents, who received a percentage of the premium income collected, had a strong financial incentive to admit such contributors, and by this method individuals who would have failed a friendly society or other medical examination were able to obtain the services of a doctor (BMA, CPR, 1905, p. 10). By 1905, however, the role of the insurance companies was being reduced due to pressure exerted through the General Medical Council (BMA, CPR, p. 9). A district medical officer in Birmingham told the Royal Commission on the Poor Laws that before the GMC's advertising and canvassing bans there had been a great many commercial and private clubs. Because of the GMC rulings these had been driven out of existence (RCPL, 1909, Appendix IV, Q. 43998(43)).

Fourth, there were the self-organized medical clubs.

Membership of the Friendly Societies

Membership figures for registered friendly societies are published annually by the Registrar of Friendly Societies. But in some years the total figure includes 'collecting societies' which were more like industrial assurance companies than friendly societies proper and invariably offered only a death benefit. To arrive at the membership of friendly societies offering a full range of services – specifically sick pay, funeral benefit, and medical care – the membership of the collecting societies has to be deducted.

After adjustment downwards to exclude the collecting societies the official figure requires adjustment upwards to take into account members of unregistered friendly societies. In a paper published in 1972 Dr Charles Hanson discussed the evidence for the extent of unregistered friendly society membership. The Royal Commission on the Friendly Societies of 1874 reported, after searching inquiry, that 'the extent of unregistered societies was as large as that of registered societies'. But did this continue to be the case over the next forty years or so? Sir Edward Brabrook, the Chief Registrar of Friendly Societies, testified to the Royal Commission on Labour of 1893 that the ratio of registered to unregistered members was still about the same. There were 3.8 million registered friendly society members out of an industrial male population of 7 million. Allowing for double membership this represented at least 3 million individuals in registered societies, and assuming a similar number of unregistered members there were at least 6 million members in total. In addition, Brabrook felt that some trade union members should also be added to the total, for some trade unions also offered friendly benefits. And we know that trade unions were in competition with the friendly societies for members, at least to some extent. In Newcastle upon Tyne in 1907, for example, trade unions were tending to offer sick pay more frequently with the result that some friendly societies lost members due to their reluctance to pay both trade union and friendly society contributions (RCPL, 1909, Appendix V, Q. 52127). In 1893 there were about 870,000 trade union members. Some of these should be added to Brabrook's 6 million. Brabrook concluded: 'It would look as if there was really merely a kind of residuum left of those who are in uncertain work or otherwise, and are not able to insure in some shape or other' (RCL, 1893, Fourth Report, Minutes of Evidence (sitting as a whole), Qs 1331–2). He confirmed his view two years later before the Royal Commission on the Aged Poor. A member of his staff had recently visited Norfolk and found many unregistered societies. In many cases some old registered societies of a hundred years standing or more had been replaced by unregistered societies: 'So I think it beyond doubt that the sphere of unregistered societies is exceedingly large' (RCAP, 1895, Q. 11039).

Can this assumption still be made on the eve of National Insurance to enable an estimate to be made of those covered by friendly societies for medical care? Giving evidence to the Royal Commission on the Poor Laws in 1906 Brabrook was still confident of his judgement that unregistered membership was about equal to registered membership. But in earlier evidence he was testifying about coverage for sick pay. His evidence to the Royal Commission on the Poor Laws concerned persons covered for *any* kind of benefit. He thought there were probably 14 million persons in unregistered societies, but half would have been infants. He put the total registered and unregistered membership at 20 million at least, allowing for double counting (RCPL, 1909, Appendix III, Qs 35147(7), 35174–80).

We also have the evidence presented to the Royal Commission by A.C. Kay and H.V. Toynbee. They carried out a major investigation of voluntary provision for the poor in several towns and rural areas. They studied three large towns (Norwich, York, and Coventry), two moderate-sized towns (Beverley and Kendal), three small towns (Ludlow, Lichfield, and Bourne), and five rural districts. Brabrook had referred to the 'growing popularity' of slate clubs (ibid., Appendix III, Q. 35147(10)), and Kay and Toynbee certainly found a large number of unregistered dividing societies in the areas they investigated. They found that dividing societies were commonly attached to public houses and workplaces in York, Norwich and Coventry. There was an especially large one at Coleman's in Norwich, and 'nearly all' the Coventry factories had dividing societies. In York they were attached to the Adult Schools. Some were attached to churches, but to a far smaller extent than they believed to have been the case in earlier years (RCPL, Appendix XIV, pp. 106, 134, 157; but cf. Rowntree, 1901, pp. 357–64). In the moderate-sized towns studied, Beverley and Kendal, they also found unregistered works clubs or friendly societies (ibid., pp. 167, 175). In the three small towns there was some variation. In Lichfield there was a dividing society but no figures are given. In Bourne there were 280 members of registered friendly societies, and 140 members of one unregistered friendly society, plus ninety members of the Bourne Self-Aiding Medical Club, and an unknown membership of 'several' dividing societies (ibid., pp. 185, 197). At Cullompton (in Devon) there were 166 members of registered societies, an unregistered dividing society with 130 members, and a works club with fifty members at a local lace factory (ibid., p. 202). They found few unregistered dividing societies in the five rural districts studied, although an unregistered society was prominent in Fairford (in Gloucestershire) and there was a small society in Little Walsingham (in Norfolk) (ibid., p. 210).

Brabrook's figure of 20 million is not satisfactory for the present purpose of estimating how many persons were covered for medical care. Beveridge calculated that about 4.75 million were members of registered societies offering sick pay in 1910 (1948, p. 76). This figure can safely be doubled to arrive at the total registered and unregistered membership of friendly societies paying sick pay. Of this 9.5 million persons, a few would not have been covered for medical care, but the vast majority were. This means that at least 9 million of the 12 million originally included in the National Insurance scheme were already members of friendly societies offering medical care.

Beveridge's 4.75 million appears to exclude members of death and burial societies who did not pay sick pay. But some did employ doctors on contract terms. A burial club at Macclesfield was one such case (*BMJ*, 18 June 1904, p. 1458). The figure also excludes those in specialized friendly societies, which again did not offer sick pay. But among these were the medical societies or medical institutes which did employ doctors. Membership was 329,450 in 1910 (Beveridge, 1948, p. 331). Most were members of friendly societies and will therefore already have been counted, but some were not. The estimate of 4.75 million members of unregistered societies includes those in works clubs. In 1911 there were just over a million miners. In colliery districts we know that medical care was provided through works clubs. Membership comprised not only miners but also steelworkers and employees of other factories operating in colliery areas. The 4.75 million therefore includes well over a million in mining areas alone, not counting miners' families, who were also covered.

Titmuss concluded that 'many of the wage-earning population, small shopkeepers and a substantial proportion of the middle-classes' received medical care through contract practice (1959, p. 306). He may have overstated middle-class membership, but the evidence otherwise suggests that about three quarters of those eventually insured under the 1911 scheme were already covered by insurance schemes before the Act was passed. The remainder either paid private fees or sought care from the charities or voluntary hospitals.

Did the Poor Join Friendly Societies?
Rowntree found in York in 1901 that the '*very poor* are but seldom members of Friendly Societies', and he commented that, 'Even if they can be induced to join, they soon allow their membership to lapse' (1901, p. 357n.; emphasis in original). In this section I will consider whether, from the patchy evidence available, this applied elsewhere. I will also examine the related point of view, sometimes expressed in modern histories used as textbooks, that the friendly societies catered only for the well-paid workers. Gilbert writes, for example, that the friendly societies 'made no appeal whatever to the grey, faceless, lower third of the working-class':

Friendly society membership was the badge of the skilled worker. Some of the societies, for instance the Hearts of Oak, maintained a minimum income limit. . . Friendly society membership was not for the crossing sweeper, the dock labourer, the railroad navvy, any more than it was for the landowner, the member of Parliament, or the company director (1966, pp. 166–7).

The overwhelming majority of the friendly societies did not maintain an income limit, including the largest and most successful societies. Indeed, they were opposed to any such distinction as a matter of principle. And in the case of the Hearts of Oak, its official 24s a week income limit had been 'abrogated' in practice (Rothschild, 1898, Appendix H, p. 154, para. 16). But this is not the only reason for suspecting that Gilbert overstates the case.

Many dock workers were in shop (works) clubs run by the dock companies, usually on dividing principles. But some were also in the permanent friendly societies. This was demonstrated in 1898 when the London and East India Docks Company tried to forbid employees from being members of outside societies. The company had organized its own Docks Friendly Society to pay sick pay. They found that men who belonged to an outside friendly society as well as to the company society had an inducement to stay off work, because the company sick pay plus the outside sick pay came to more than their own wage. When membership of outside friendly societies was banned Manchester Unity and the other large societies campaigned vigorously against it. They pressed parliament for legislation to forbid companies from restricting their employees' freedom of choice in this manner, arguing that there was a parallel with 'truck', the system of payment in kind (*Oddfellows Magazine*, February 1898, pp. 40–46; April 1901, pp. 103–4).

This shows two things. First that there were some dock workers in the large friendly societies, certainly enough to alarm their leaders when the company forced its employees to leave. Secondly, it shows that the friendly societies were keen to recruit from among dock workers. So if the dockers did not join, it was not the doing of the large friendly societies. Testimony to the Royal Commission on the Poor Laws also tends to contradict Gilbert. The Royal Commission was told that among the 4,000 Manchester Unity members in Liverpool were a 'good many' earning irregular wages averaging less than 25s a week. Many of these were dock workers, but generally the Royal Commission was told that dock workers belonged to their own dividing societies (RCPL, 1909, Appendix IV, Qs 37377–84). Finally, evidence from Huddersfield suggests that low-paid railway labourers joined the major friendly societies in large numbers. A Huddersfield Poor Law guardian who was also a member of the Ancient Order of Foresters, testified that a 'large majority' of local AOF members were unskilled labourers such as railway labourers earning 18s a week. Indeed, the 'vast majority' of railwaymen, including the lowest paid, joined both friendly societies and trade unions. Some earned even less, but most unskilled workers in Huddersfield earned from 18s to 22s 6d a week (ibid., Appendix IV, Qs. 41792–800). Manchester Unity members' wage rates were also reported to start from the 18s mark, rising to 28s a week (ibid., Appendix IV, Appendix LII (2)).

Kay and Toynbee's investigation revealed that in the three large towns they studied wage rates were lowest in Norwich, with skilled workers earning as little as 20s a week rising to 30s, and unskilled workers earning from 18s to 23s. Yet in Norwich, friendly society membership was much higher than in the other towns. Friendly society leaders told the investigators that this was *because* wages were low: the lower paid had to think more carefully about how to provide for themselves in the event of sickness. Better paid workers had more alternatives available (RCPL, 1909, Appendix XIV, pp. 106–7). The investigators found this surprising and pursued the issue further. Generally they found that registered friendly society membership was highest in rural areas where wages were lowest. They repro-duced a table which had been published by the Ancient Order of Foresters (the second largest society) comparing AOF member-ship in 1902 with county populations in 1901. Rural counties scored highest, and the industrialized ones the lowest.

TABLE 3 **AOF Membership in Rural Counties**

County	Members per 1000 population
Norfolk	61.37
Suffolk	49.69
Bedfordshire	48.42
Shropshire	47.45
Northamptonshire	44.88
Herefordshire	43.96
Hertfordshire	43.54
Wiltshire	42.49
Dorsetshire	41.31

The Norfolk figure of 61.37 per 1000 was the highest, and Lanca-shire, a highly industrialized county, was lowest with 3.82 (ibid., p. 107). Other evidence from industrialized Coventry suggested that when workers earned higher wages they turned to other forms of investment like saving (ibid., p. 157).

The investigators were not the only ones to be surprised by the figures. J.L. Stead, the permanent secretary of the AOF, said he had been astounded that some of their best branches were in areas with the lowest wages and that they were weakest in the larger towns where wages were high (RCPL, 1909, Appendix VII, Qs. 77557–8). He thought that the membership of the other permanent friendly societies was similar, and expressed his pride in the fact that they had low-paid members: 'We have got some of the humblest men in the country in our society, and we are just as proud of them as of the others' (ibid., Qs 77543–4).

The Royal Commission received a good deal of other testimony on the availability of medical clubs to the poor. In Somerset, for instance, club members were reported to be largely mechanics, but there were also many among the 'labouring classes' (RCPL, 1909, Appendix vol. VII, appendix LXI (5)). In Yeovil the former medical officer of health said that medical clubs were within the reach of all but the 'very poorest' (ibid., appendix LXI (10–11)). Another witness told the commission that in Somerset the 'younger, better class' of agricultural labourers belonged mostly to the permanent friendly societies, whilst older men tended to belong to the (less reliable) annual dividing societies (ibid., appendix XXIII(5)).

According to a district medical officer in Oxford, the 'great majority' of the 'respectable poor' did join clubs or provident dispensaries (RCPL, 1909, Appendix III, Q. 34123). But Percy Alden, MP, told the royal commission that unskilled workers in his locality tended not to join medical clubs, preferring to attend a 'cheap doctor', who charged 6d a visit (ibid., Qs 27901, 27906).

There is other indirect evidence that clubs catered for the poor. Sir William Chance, MP, told the Royal Commission that whenever a medical aid association was established pauperism diminished (Appendix III, Q. 27061(56)). In Liverpool there were a great many 'sixpenny dispensaries' which charged, as the name implies, 6d for each consultation, including medicine. A large number of the 'lower working class' sought treatment in these dispensaries. And, the Commission were told, some very poor persons preferred to save up the 6d required rather than seek Poor Law assistance (Appendix IV, Qs 38324(5)). Also in Liverpool there were a great many unregistered friendly societies known locally as tontines. The Royal Commission were told that 'nearly all' doctors in Liverpool served the tontines (Appendix IV, Q. 38325). The usual medical contribution was 4s a year, sometimes 3s (ibid., Q. 38324(2)). In Manchester, however, the medical officer of health said he had been informed that friendly society members did not earn less than 30s a week. But the fact that his evidence was second hand vitiates it somewhat (RCPL, Appendix IV, Qs 38380(55), 38390).

A Northampton doctor complained to the GMC that from the whole population of Northampton: 'You can scarcely get a private fee. Excepting the richest manufacturers, wealthiest tradesmen, and professional men, they are all members of some Dispensary or similar organization.' The Royal Victoria Dispensary had four medical officers, the Friendly Societies Medical Institute had three medical officers plus a dispenser, in addition to which there was the Homoeopathic Dispensary which charged 2s 6d a month. Every local doctor except the four Infirmary staff had clubs (GMC, 1893, pp. 39–40). In his view: 'It is inexpressibly sad and degrading that men of education and refinement should be at the mercy of combinations of low insurance agents, petty tradesmen, mechanics, and others' (GMC, 1893, p. 39).

A district medical officer in Northampton confirmed that medical clubs were very common, and reported that there was a feeling against the Poor Law among those he described as the 'better class poor'. A district medical officer in Sheffield expressed a similar view (RCPL, 1909, Appendix vol. IV, Q. 47921(11); appendix LXXXIII(16)).

According to the Northumberland county medical officer of health, in both Newcastle upon Tyne and the country districts there were many medical clubs, and 'all the miners and many, if not most of the workmen' were members. The poor turned partly to the Poor Law and partly to the Newcastle Dispensary, and to some extent to the Royal Victoria Infirmary and the specialist hospitals (the Eye Infirmary, the Children's Hospital, the Throat and Ear Hospital, and the Hospital for Diseases of the Skin). But the voluntary hospitals catered as much for the better off as for the poor (RCPL, 1909, Appendix vol. IV, appendix LXXXIII(5)).

Other evidence confirms that many workers on low wages

joined the leading friendly societies. Claverhouse Graham, president of the Old Age State Pensions League, a director of Manchester Unity since 1890, and an advocate of old age pensions, told a select committee of the House of Commons that the friendly societies did not only recruit the highest paid workers. The lowest paid were members too. In the Eastern counties agricultural labourers on 14s to 15s a week were members. And he reckoned the average wage of members of all the societies was not one pound a week, at a time when the national average was much more (SCADP, 1899, Qs 1701–2).

There was quite a large turnover of friendly society members, but according to the AOF in Huddersfield those that tended to come and go were in the eighteen to thirty age group (RCPL, 1909, Appendix IV, Q. 41804; Appendix VII, Q. 77538). This was also the view of the Chief Registrar of Friendly Societies (RCAP, 1895, Qs 11236–7). But many of those who joined, left, and rejoined were receiving low wages, or were affected by the trade cycle. In Sheffield, for instance, the Royal Commission was told that men who could not keep up their contributions eventually joined the dividing societies (Appendix IV, Qs 43219–20; see also BMA, CPR, p.7).

The dividing societies did not have the stability of the affiliated orders, and offered less security. But they were keen to improve their services, and prepared to band together to do so. For example, for those members who lived too far from their own society's local base to use the society medical officer a scheme was introduced in 1908 to give them a choice among the medical officers of other dividing societies. It was organized by the Federated Societies Medical Benefit Scheme, which was to arrange for about a hundred doctors to form a panel from which members could choose (*BMJ*, 13 February 1909, p. 425).

To sum up: there are no suitable statistics which enable a precise estimate of the number of persons on low incomes who joined friendly societies to be made. The chief evidence is the testimony of contemporary observers and investigators. From this evidence it can reasonably be inferred that a considerable number of poor persons did join friendly societies, including the large national federations. Many others did not join. From this it follows that having a low income or few material resources did not, alone, determine whether or not a person joined a friendly society. The beliefs and attitudes – the culture – of each poor person played its part. Moreover, there is no indication that the friendly societies actively deterred the poor from joining – indeed, they were proud to have them. But there were many who ranked among the low paid, and particularly those with irregular or seasonal earnings, who found it hard to keep up the contributions. Here was a group which needed assistance.

Were Other Groups Excluded from Contract Practice?
'Speaking broadly', the Minority Report of the Royal Commission on the Poor Laws of 1909 found that the friendly societies did not provide medical attendance 'for any woman, whether married or single, or for children'. And the friendly societies 'do not, if they can help it, admit "bad lives", against which all friendly societies protect themselves by a medical examination prior to admission, or any person suffering from constitutional defects, or incipient disease.' Nor did they provide for existing members who suffered from venereal disease or were ill due to alcoholic excess. In the judgement of the Minority Report, these excluded classes amounted to 'more than three fourths of the population' (RCPL, MR, 1909, p. 870). Some modern studies have also emphasized that contract practice was not available to women and children. Describing the situation before 1911, Levitt writes that contract practice was 'only available to the wage earner himself – wives, children, the old and disabled had to rely on outpatient departments and dispensaries of the voluntary hospitals or *go without*' (Levitt, 1977, p. 13; emphasis added).

The claim that some people had to go without altogether is wrong. Some kind of medical care was available to everyone, even if it was only the Poor Law. No one at all went without, unless by choice. However, contract practice – which does not include outpatient departments, charitable dispensaries, or the Poor Law – was not available to everyone.

Friendly societies did usually require that new members should enjoy good health. Earlier in the last century, a medical examination had sometimes been compulsory and sometimes not, although by the last quarter of the century it was a requirement in the vast majority of societies. In the Ancient Order of

Foresters in 1857, for instance, the decision whether or not to require a medical examination had been at the discretion of branches. Some had required an examination and some had not. However, by 1907, an examination was compulsory (*General Laws*, 1857, rule 65; 1907, rule 38). But it is unwise to take the requirements laid down in friendly society rulebooks as a necessary reflection of what actually happened. And in the case of the medical examination there was considerable laxity. Whether or not many people were excluded by the medical examination varied greatly. Much depended on the medical officer. Some were strict; others were not.

A doctor in Kent pointed out that he was 'well satisfied' with his club practice, and attributed this to the fact that he carried out a strict medical examination. He said he knew of 'many' doctors who were 'slack' in this respect and so faced a higher workload (BMA, CPR, 1905, p. 44). But some of the small friendly societies carried out strict medicals. The Ideal Benefit Society, for example, was said to carry out 'very careful' medicals (RCPL, Appendix IV, Q. 44875). Local dividing societies were usually very lax and often had no medical. However, there is evidence from one source that some local dividing societies, which members joined afresh every year, would exclude sick members at the annual meeting (BMA, CPR, 1905, p. 18).

The medical officer of the Bradford Friendly Societies Medical Association was strict about medicals. He rejected 197 out of 641 candidates in 1887, and 11 out of 400 in 1888 (Bradford FSMA, *Annual Report*, 1888). In 1882 the medical officer of the Nottingham Friendly Societies Medical Institution rejected 46 out of 358 candidates; in 1883 32 out of 470; in 1884 19 out of 471; and in 1885, 11 out of 1,022 (*Annual Reports*). Overall this represents a rejection rate of about 4½ per cent. But medical officers who were strict could not afford to exceed the standards prevailing in the society that employed them. If they did they were likely to be replaced. Most friendly societies were keen to recruit, and if friends or relatives could be 'got in' despite the formal rule, so much the better. For example, at the turn of the century, according to the *Lancet*, the Ancient Order of Foresters was very anxious to recruit members and as a result their admission procedures were very lax (*Lancet*, 7 April 1900, p. 1033). In other cases it was not necessary to obtain a certificate from the branch medical officer. Some societies accepted a certificate from any qualified doctor (BMA, CPR, 1905, p. 16).

Formally the Hearts of Oak was one of the most strict societies. In 1892 the 175,000-strong society, one of the centralized friendly societies which was expanding rapidly in the 1890s, excluded by rule all those earning less than 24s a week and men in 'unhealthy or dangerous' trades. But according to evidence given to the Rothschild committee of 1898, these rules had in practice been 'abrogated' (Appendix H, p. 154, para. 16). Hearts of Oak did not offer medical benefit, although many of its members did establish local clubs to employ doctors. As early as 1871 members had formed such clubs in seventy-three different localities (Gosden, 1961, p. 141).

A number of persons, therefore, were excluded from friendly society membership by the medical examination. That is, they were excluded from some societies, for there was a simple way of avoiding the requirement of good health. This was to join a temperance friendly society. The proselytizing zeal of these societies led some to accept nearly anyone into the fold, healthy or not (see e.g. RCPL, 1909, Appendix vol. V, appendix CI(35)). This was, perhaps, one reason for the sustained growth of the Rechabites, the largest of the teetotal societies. In 1910 they had over 317,000 members.

In the 1890s and subsequently the main group experiencing difficulty in obtaining medical care on contract terms, in some areas at least, was women. This was due, not to the policy of the friendly societies, but to the doctors. Some doctors had refused to take women on contract terms from the earliest days of club practice. Manchester Unity's Clarence Lodge in Brighton, for instance, appointed its first surgeon in 1830 at a penny a week per member. The following year the surgeon announced that he intended to decline to 'attend females' at contract rates (District Annals and Guide, Brighton AMC, 1911, pp. 45, 47).

Many doctors continued to refuse to serve women on club terms. When the United Sisters Friendly Society was founded attempts to establish branches in several towns foundered on the refusal of doctors to cooperate. At Newton-on-Trent lodge surgeons 'would have nothing' of the proposed branch. They would only agree to carry out medical examinations (for a very high fee). Their view, expressed with 'almost brutal frankness', was that it was bad enough having to attend men on club terms, but if they had to attend women too, they would be unable to make a living (*Oddfellows Magazine*, April 1889, p. 118). In 1900 doctors at Skipton refused to supply medical attendance to a proposed female lodge (*Oddfellows Magazine*, May 1900, p. 145). And friendly societies at Barnstaple had a similar experience (*Oddfellows Magazine*, September 1900, p. 388).

However in some friendly society lodges it was possible for women to pay for medical attendance. For example in the Wisbech lodges 191 females (some wives and some widows) paid for medical attendance in 1890. Total membership was 975. In addition there had also been since 1885 an official female lodge with thirty members (*Oddfellows Magazine*, June 1890, pp. 169–70). By the 1890s this was becoming more and more common. And by 1905 the BMA were complaining that, due to the tendency of women to join clubs, contract practice was losing its attraction as a means of introduction to potential patients (BMA, CPR, 1905, p. 17). Some Manchester Unity and AOF branches offered family terms. Manchester Unity's St George's Lodge in Leeds, for example, preferred to employ its own doctor instead of using the medical institute. Fees were: adults, 3s; juveniles, 2s; family, 10s 6d (RCPL, Appendix IV, Q. 41489(18)).

However, in many districts doctors successfully refused to serve women on club terms up to the eve of National Insurance. The Royal Commission on the Poor Laws was told that the Newcastle Medico-Ethical Society was continuing to successfully boycott female lodges (Appendix vol. V, appendix CI(25–6)). And in 1907, in the Ancient Order of Foresters, only a 'rather low' percentage of branches offered family cover (ibid., Appendix VII, Q. 77431).

In districts where works clubs were available – mainly mining districts – women and children were covered (BMA, CPR, 1905, p. 8). And in such localities the ordinary friendly societies sometimes offered family cover. In Swansea, for example, family rates in 1907 were 8s 8d, increased about three years earlier from 6s (RCPL, Appendix V, Q. 50856(23–4)). Usually no medical examination was required to obtain the doctor's services. There were in 1911, 1,067,213 miners in the United Kingdom. They must have had at least 3 million dependants, and probably nearer 4 million. Allowing for non-mining members, it is not unreasonable to suppose that at least 4 million women and children were covered by colliery works clubs alone.

Why did doctors refuse on such a large scale to serve women on contract terms? It was not because they were women as such, but because doctors believed that it was more costly to attend females. Women were regarded as more vulnerable to sickness (a belief reflected in the administration of the 1911 National Insurance scheme). As a result doctors preferred to charge a fee for each attendance, or, if they were willing to contemplate contract cover, they sought a higher annual contribution than was customary for males. Given the wide availability of free medical care in the voluntary hospitals, there was a strong reluctance on the part of the friendly societies to pay higher rates for women members.

To sum up: the evidence indicates that on the eve of National Insurance, many women and children in many localities were not able to obtain medical care on contract terms. But gradually contract practice was being extended, and more particularly, the growth of medical institutes (which provided for the whole family) was rapid. Works club provided for still more dependants. However, from the patchy evidence available, I conclude that a majority of women and children would have been unable to obtain contract cover if they had wanted it. This was either because doctors would not offer it, or because there was no local medical institute or works club. Women and children turned to the outpatient departments of the hospitals, or consulted private doctors for a fee.

6
Compulsory National Insurance: The Immediate Impact

The government proposal for National Insurance, first published in 1910, brought about a swift change in the attitude of the profession. In 1903 contract practice had been described by the *BMJ* as in theory economically sound and 'in some forms . . . one of the pleasantest ways in which a medical man can earn his living' (*BMJ*, 6 January 1903, p. 1339). But in a leading article in 1910 the *BMJ* argued that the prospect of compulsory sickness insurance had created a new situation:

> In fact it comes to this – that, under compulsory sickness insurance, if contract practice is to be acquiesced in at all, it will have to be accepted on a vastly bigger scale than at present. The Association will therefore have to face without delay the question whether it is not possible and infinitely preferable for all parties concerned, doctors and patients alike, altogether to abolish contract practice. . . (*BMJ*, 25 June 1910, p. 1561).

As one doctor put it, with compulsory state insurance the *raison d'etre* of contract practice had gone: 'We now resume our place as medical practitioners pure and simple, ready as sellers to give our service to the buyer, who is now not the poverty-stricken wage earner, but the solvent State Insurance Company.' Once the state became involved the willingness of some doctors to act according to once unchallenged moral principles declined. Capitation payment was to be ruled out because this maintained the burden of responsibility on the doctor, a responsibility they had accepted before government intervention, but would not accept after it. Payment for work done was the only acceptable method. Arguing against a colleague who held that doctors should continue to be willing to carry the risk of 'the yearly variation of sickness', the correspondent asked why the profession should meet the risk of an epidemic 'out of its own pocket, health and strength'. Doctors now dealt with 'a solvent state instead of with an insolvent patient'. The state should pay the full cost (*BMJ*, 12 November 1910, p. 1556). Doctors felt strongly that conditions they had accepted in the marketplace should not be imposed on them by the state (see e.g. *BMJ*, 12 November 1910, pp. 1557–8). And in particular, they saw their chance to get rid of lay control (*BMJ*, 12 November 1910, p. 1559).

Doctors have often been seen as arch-enemies of state intervention, an impression reinforced by their vigorous initial opposition to the government plan. But the disagreement was about the terms, it was not about the principle of a state takeover. Indeed medical opinion had been, albeit slowly, growing in sympathy for state medicine for some years (see e.g. *BMJ*, 4 July 1896, p. 10).

Did the 1911 National Insurance Act strengthen or weaken the power of the medical consumer? Or did it increase the power of the medical profession at the expense of the consumer? The fixing of capitation fees for insured persons was taken out of the marketplace, with the result that medical incomes doubled. The self-governing organizations of manual workers were pushed aside and the power to organize the new medical benefit given to bodies heavily under the influence of the medical profession. The 1911 Act also granted registered medical practitioners a monopoly on panel practice. The 1858 Medical Act, the main legislation regulating the medical profession, had not granted registered practitioners such a wide-ranging monopoly. Persons not licensed by the medical licensing authorities, such as homoeopathists, naturopaths, and so on, could and did practice medicine. But under the 1911 Act, only registered practitioners could become panel doctors. The twelve million insured persons, many of whom had turned to unqualified persons before the Act, were therefore denied the freedom to spend their incomes in that manner. According to a government survey of 1910, there were large numbers of unqualified persons practising medicine and enjoying the confidence of the public (PMSUP, 1910). The 1911 Act helped to drive them out of business. It was reinforced by the 1920 Dangerous Drugs Act, which prohibited all but registered medical practitioners from possessing certain drugs essential to medical practice; and by the Venereal Diseases Act of 1917 which prohibited all but registered medical practitioners from treating venereal disease.

Control

Under the Act control of the medical benefit – medical attendance supplied by a panel doctor plus the medicines prescribed – was taken from the friendly societies and passed to insurance committees. What was the position of the medical profession within the apparatus administering medical benefit? In England and Wales there was a local insurance committee for every county and county borough. Three fifths of the members were elected by insured persons, one fifth by the local authority, and of the remaining fifth two were elected by the medical profession, one was a doctor appointed by the local authority and the remainder were appointed by the Ministry of Health.

The insurance committee had to confer with three other committees: the local medical committee, representing all doctors in the area; the local panel committee, representing all panel doctors in the area (often identical with the medical committee); and the local pharmaceutical committee, representing local chemists. The insurance committee also had a medical service sub-committee consisting of an equal number of professional representatives and insured persons. The chairman and vice-chairman were drawn from those members of the insurance committee nominated by the local authority or the Ministry of Health who were neither doctors nor insured persons. The sub-committee investigated all complaints made against doctors.

Representation on these bodies gave the profession greatly enhanced power, compared with the situation before 1911. But it was not their representation locally that was decisive. Notwithstanding the formally decentralized administration of the scheme, power at the centre was very great. And here the BMA was strongly represented, and extremely influential. The insurance commission, later the Ministry of Health, could not recognize the BMA as representative of the whole medical profession, but this was overcome by means of the BMA's Insurance Acts Committee which was recognized by the Ministry of Health. It was made up of thirty-seven members, five *ex officio*, five elected by the Representative Body, twenty-three by local medical and panel committees, and four by other bodies. The members of the local medical and panel committees may not have been BMA members. The machinery was frequently used, especially in the 1920s when the doctors' rate of pay was in dispute.

Besides lobbying through its place in official machinery the BMA continued to function as a trade union, pursuing its aims by the use of techniques like black listing. It refused to accept advertisements for positions of which it disapproved, or when it disliked the rate of pay, and issued warning notices about non-approved positions. In the 1920s the BMA blacklisted some local authorities who would not pay BMA rates for salaried medical officers, such as medical officers of health or school medical officers. Their methods succeeded, for example, in preventing the Worcester County Council from securing a suitable assistant county medical officer (Carr-Saunders and Wilson, 1933, p. 99).

The government took away power from the autonomous clubs and handed it to the insurance committees because Lloyd George seems to have wholly accepted the doctors' case. In the House of Commons on 29 May he said:

> One of the most important professions in the land is treated in a way which, I think, is perfectly disgraceful to those who have arranged such terms of payment, and not only discreditable, but stupid. I cannot imagine how they could expect the best services from doctors who are paid at that rate. . . The doctor . . . whom the club might starve out of existence if he dared to refuse them – has been driven to accepting 2s 6d for members, including drugs.

In future, he announced, the BMA would make its representations to the Health Commission, not the friendly societies. In a speech to the BMA on 2 June he announced the 'absolute control' by the friendly societies was 'at an end forever under the Bill'. He also accused the friendly societies of making a profit out of the doctors by saving money that ought to go to the doctors and using it for other benefits: 'It will be part of our responsibility,' Lloyd George announced, 'to see that the money which we intend shall go for medical benefits shall go there, and shall not go into the pockets of friendly societies for distribution or any other benefits' (*Oddfellows Magazine*, July 1911, p. 350).

This was an entirely wrong interpretation of the situation. The average fee was over 4s, not 2s 6d. The BMA had found in 1905 that only about 8 per cent of doctors were being paid 3s or less. The non-profit friendly societies were particularly stung by the accusation that they made a profit. Some members felt that contract practice, in some localities at least, was 'money for old rope'. Far from the friendly societies profiting from club practice, one delegate told the Manchester Unity's annual conference in 1911, there was a saying in his locality that friendly society medical contributions went to pay for greasing the doctors' carriage wheels (*Oddfellows Magazine*, July 1911, p. 350). And no friendly society did make a profit. In lodge practice the whole of the members' contribution was usually paid to the doctors. And in the case of medical aid associations, if surpluses were accumulated they were always ploughed back into the medical service in the form of improved buildings, extra help in epidemics and so on.

The loss of control of the medical benefit meant that the friendly societies lost the protection their rulebooks gave them. The range of services was now a matter for the government; and complaints about doctors were to be handled by committees on which doctors were strongly represented. Friendly society members were proud of their independence and felt the loss of their medical service keenly. The Act was seen by the *Oddfellows Magazine* as an attempt to deny the working class the right to self-government:

> Working men are awakening to the fact that this is a subtle attempt to take from the class to which they belong the administration of the great voluntary organizations which they have built up for themselves, and to hand over the future control to the paid servants of the governing class. . . This is not liberty; this is not development of self-government, but a new form of autocracy and tyranny not less but the more dangerous because it is benevolent in its intentions (*Oddfellows Magazine*, September 1911, p. 544).

And the High Chief Ranger of the Foresters warned the Chancellor at their annual conference in 1911 that he was in danger of robbing 'the working classes of all right of free association' (AOF, *Quarterly Reports*, 1911, p. 82).

In a leading article, the *Oddfellows Magazine* described the medical benefit decision as 'an insult to the working-class population of the country':

> To say, as the Bill now says, to the working class of the United Kingdom, 'You must be compelled, every one of you who earns less than £160 a year, to pay for medical attendance in case of sickness, but you are unfit to be entrusted with the administration of your own money; you are a lot of sweaters, you have cruelly treated a great profession, and so we will administer the money for you through committees, on which the medical officer who is to be paid with your money shall be represented so that he may fix both his remuneration and the measure of his service', is not merely an unbusinesslike proposition, but a flagrant insult to every working man and woman in the land. Why should working men and women be degraded to an inferior position? (*Oddfellows Magazine*, September 1911, pp. 544–5).

Pay

The leading complaint voiced by the doctors before the 1911 Act was that they were underpaid. As a result of the government scheme they secured a very large increase in their incomes. But this did not stem the tide of complaint. Doctors' complaints about low fees – so often taken at face value by critics of pre-1911 health care – did not stop with the acceptance of the Act. After 1911 they were directed at government instead of the friendly societies. Initially the government had offered the doctors 6s per insured patient, including medicine. This was a generous offer, for the minimum contract practice rate then being demanded by the BMA was 5s, itself higher than some market rates. In February 1912 the BMA demanded 8s 6d, excluding medicine. A survey of doctors' incomes was carried out by Sir William Plender, who was asked to visit six towns – three to be selected by the Insurance Commission and three by the BMA – to ascertain the charges being made for medical treatment.

Sir William studied the income of doctors in 1910 and 1911 in Cardiff, Darlington, Darwen, Dundee, Norwich and St Albans. He approached 265 doctors, of whom fifty-one refused access to their records. Forty of the fifty-one were in Cardiff, and for this reason Cardiff was dropped from the study.

Sir William reported in July that in the remaining five towns, the average annual gross income of doctors in private practice, less a proportion for bad debts, was 4s 2d per patient. If income from contract patients was added, the average worked out at 4s 1¾d. The average annual capitation fee being paid was 3s 11d. The average of 4s 2d requires adjustment because Dundee doctors did not dispense medicines. In an estimate prepared by the Insurance Commission for England, 4s 5d was suggested as a more accurate figure, allowing for the cost of medicines in Dundee (Plender, 1912; ICE, 1912–13, p. 128).

The *British Medical Journal* immediately denounced Plender's findings as biased and incorrect, and the BMA continued to press for an increase in the 6s being offered. The government responded by raising its offer to 7s 6d. This was also rejected. On 23 October the government finally raised its offer to 9s 0d (including medicines). This offer was also rejected by the BMA.

By this time, however, rifts were beginning to appear within the medical profession. The leadership of the BMA was out of touch with the rank and file, who knew only too well that acceptance of 9s 0d would mean the near doubling of their incomes. In January 1913 the 9s 0d offer was accepted.

Some doctors opposed payment by capitation fee altogether, and for this reason insurance committees were entitled to adopt alternative methods of payment. In fact, only three areas – Manchester, Salford, and Kent – adopted the fee-for-service method of payment, and in Kent it was abandoned within a year. It was maintained in the other areas for some years, but eventually quietly dropped (ICE, 1912–13, pp. 147–8).

Soon after the war the capitation fee again became controversial. In March 1920 doctors had been granted 11s 0d by an arbitrator after claiming 13s 6d. They accepted the decision but continued to regard 11s 0d as 'inadequate to cover the services rendered' (*Oddfellows Magazine*, October 1921, p. 534). The government then sought a reduction in the fee as part of its package of economy measures. Sir Alfred Mond, the minister of health, reminded the doctors, as his predecessor Addison had done, that they were financially much better off than they had been in the market: 'I am sure that you do not wish to escape from the Scylla of the Ministry of Health to the Charybdis of the friendly societies' (Eder, 1982, p. 125). In January 1922 the capitation fee was reduced to 9s 6d. Then in late 1923 the Ministry of

Health proposed a reduction to 8s 6d for three years or 8s for five years. In October 1923 a conference representing all the approved societies was held. It had objected to the pay increase the Ministry of Health proposed to award the doctors, because it would deprive insured persons of 'money which would otherwise be available for those essential benefits of a preventive and curative character, such as hospital, convalescent home, dental and optical treatment, nursing etc,' to which they were entitled (*Foresters Miscellany*, November 1923, p. 604). Nevertheless, a court of inquiry was held and fixed the fee at 9s, a figure which remained in force from January 1924 until the end of 1926 (RCNHI, 1926, Appendices, p. 93; Eder, 1982, pp. 114–33).

Conclusion

In the years leading up to the 1911 Act the unity sought by many doctors was certainly lacking. And arguably it is the duty of government to discourage the emergence of such unity. But, one of the chief results of the 1911 Act was that it stimulated the medical profession to unite at the expense of the consumer. Doctors organized a great campaign to transform the National Insurance scheme into one that benefited them at the expense of the medical consumers, and particularly friendly society members. As a result of their agitation between 1910 and 1912 the doctors made very considerable gains at the expense of the consumer: most notably, they freed themselves from lay control, insinuated themselves into the machinery of the state, and nearly doubled their incomes. (For a discussion of these gains, see Green, 1982.)

Once the state entered the scene, the organized profession found their ability to extract concessions at the expense of the consumer vastly increased. Compared with the marketplace the state offered greatly increased opportunities for the exercise of professional power. A brief but, for the doctors, all too common, illustration must suffice. The *Lancet* special commissioner described how difficult it was to maintain a cartel in the marketplace of the 1890s. In Hull the local medical society campaign enjoyed the backing of over 90 per cent of local doctors, but it took only two or three medical men 'to upset the whole combination'. For instance, it was agreed not to accept club appointments at below 4s and all but one doctor supported the minimum. This doctor entered into a secret agreement with local societies to work for less. As a result he secured a very large increase in his club patients. Soon, colleagues noticed his success and suspicions were aroused. One by one other doctors abandoned the minimum and payments dropped to 2s 6d. Two medical society members even started to use handbills. They were called to account for themselves before the branch, but simply resigned. However, a complaint was made to their licensing authority, and 'they were duly warned' with the result that no further handbills were issued. But the cartel was broken (*Lancet*, 16 November 1895, p. 1256). The state was no pushover, as the conflict over pay from 1920 to 1924 showed, but pay increases were far more easy to obtain than in the market.

7

Solving the Knowledge/Power Imbalance: Information Sharing Devices or Professional Hegemony

In this chapter I return to the 'ignorant consumer' thesis advanced by market failure theorists. Chapter 4 examined one of their main contentions: that consumer dominance of the pre–1911 medical market produced second-rate medical care. This chapter takes the analysis further by examining the mechanisms that enabled consumers to exercise power in the market. These mechanisms served a dual role: (a) encouraging individual doctors to defy producer cartels; and (b) functioning as information-supplying devices which enabled consumers to overcome the disadvantages ensuing from the doctors' superior knowledge.

In 1522 Henry VIII had given the Royal College of Physicians and the Universities of Oxford and Cambridge a monopoly on the practice of physic, ostensibly to protect the 'rude and credulous populace'. Does the evidence suggest that nineteenth and early twentieth century consumers were also so ignorant that, for their own good, they deserved to be deprived of the market power they exercised?

The 'Rude and Credulous Populace'
The problem for the consumer, put at its simplest, is how to select a good doctor from experience without being maimed or killed in the process. Each person's direct experience of medical practitioners may well be very limited, and so there are considerable advantages in learning from the experience of others.

Membership of an organization with a sense of brotherhood, a procedure for collective appointment of a shared medical officer, and common rules including a procedure for complaining about the doctor, was a very effective way of gaining access to a lot of other people's experience. It considerably speeded up the learning process of each individual.

To what extent was the doctor under the control of his patients? Certainly some doctors expressed strong resentment about lay control. Sometimes this resentment contained strong class overtones. According to the *Lancet* special commissioner, some years earlier the medical officer of the Northampton friendly societies' medical institute had resigned in protest at the interference of the committee, which at the time had comprised three paperhangers, three compositors, two barbers, two shoemakers, two porters, one baker, one miller, two clerks, one grocer's assistant, and an ex-policeman. This committee was said to hold in its hands 'the very conscience' of the medical officer. On one occasion when the medical officer had protested, he had been told by the committee chairman, 'You must do what we say while you *was* (sic) in our service' (emphasis in original). 'It stands to reason,' the special commissioner argued, 'that these medical servants of uneducated lay committees cannot afford to give due consideration to the welfare of the patients' (*Lancet*, 28 December 1895, pp. 1669–70).

Other doctors also resented being employed by people they looked upon as their social inferiors. One doctor complained about their condition of 'degrading bondage'. In support of his view he cited the experience of one of his assistants a few years earlier. He had been asked to have a drink with one of the coalminers for whom he acted as colliery surgeon, but had declined. The miner had been offended and retaliated, 'Ah! you're too proud to drink with me, but you're nowt but my servant, my b—— servant' (expletive deleted in original) (*BMJ*, 2 January 1909, p. 68). A colleague complained of being the 'subservient servant' of labourers and mechanics, who abused their power over the doctors because they did not know how to use it (*BMJ*, 27 November 1897, p. 1609).

Another doctor complained that a surgeon could hardly fail to 'entertain a feeling of resentment' when contract practice encouraged people to waste his time. But he added, 'If he venture to demonstrate, or if he shows haste in making the diagnosis, he will most probably receive an abusive letter from the club secretary, charging him with neglecting the members, or with failing to show them due deference.' Under such circumstances, he felt, the attitude of the doctor was likely to become 'one of indifference tempered by fear of the club secretary'. Duty to the patient was apt to be forgotten 'in his silent indignation at being sweated by a hundred ignorant and boorish taskmasters'. He called for the total abolition of contract practice (*BMJ*, 31 March 1900, p. 816).

Much of the correspondence in the medical journals showed signs of having been written by men in an agitated state of mind. An adjustment has therefore to be made for exaggeration. But, allowing for this, it is clear that the organized consumer did have some control over the way health care was delivered. How was this accomplished?

Encouraging Defiance of Producer Cartels

The underlying problem is this. It is very easy for the profession to organize against the consumer. If consumers act in the market as isolated individuals they will be weak. Given the existence of professional cartels and professional sanctions against colleagues for non-compliance, the consumer's problem is how to make it attractive for individual doctors to break cartel rates in the consumer's interests. One method is to be able to offer individual doctors sufficient guaranteed income to make it worth their while to defy their colleagues.

By banding together and electing one or more medical officers, friendly society members increased the attractiveness of their custom to a prospective doctor. Doctors did compete for individual patients by adjusting prices and service standards to suit the demands of patients. But it did not take long for doctors to calculate that they could avoid the inconvenience of competing by forming a cartel to fix minimum rates. If a doctor failed to toe the line he could be expelled from the local association, ostracized socially, denied specialist consultations, and sometimes denied access to local hospitals. Some doctors were willing to put up with the social and professional isolation in order to compete for individual patients. But the prospect of winning additional patients one by one was not enough to tempt most doctors to defy their medical brethren. The prospect of winning two or three hundred patients at once, however, was extremely inviting. One friendly society with, say, three hundred members at 4s 0d a year each would alone provide sufficient to subsist on, and four or five societies or branches would support a comfortable lifestyle. In 1907 the *BMJ* estimated the average income of GPs at between £200 and £400 (*BMJ*, 7 September 1907, p. 561; cf. 14 September 1907, p. 684).

Because of their organization in clubs, patients made it worth the while of individual doctors to defy their colleagues. Had they not been organized in clubs then each patient would have faced an organized profession as a mere individual patient who would make little difference one way or the other to the doctor's income. As I will show later, this is why doctors pressed for patients' freedom of choice. Such 'freedom' reduced the patient from being a powerful club member to being an isolated individual.

Sometimes friendly society elections took place six-monthly, sometimes annually, and sometimes doctors were elected at the pleasure of the lodge. Some elections were vigorously contested. In 1880 one doctor issued cards to lodge members:

Members of the Grange Club – Vote for Dr Warren, the poor man's friend. Vote for Dr Warren, who attends personally on you when sick. Vote for Dr Warren, who makes up his own medicines for you. Vote for Dr Warren, who, through constant and unwearying attention, saved the life of John H. Coy, when attacked with a disease which has proved so often fatal.

The chief objection of the correspondent who informed the *BMJ* about the election was that Dr Warren was drawing attention to the differences between his methods and those of his competitor, notably that he dispensed his own medicines (*BMJ*, 24 July 1880, p. 157).

This is how elections were conducted in one country district of England in 1904. Three doctors applied for a post. The oldest personally canvassed all the members for several weeks before the election making special mention of his large family. On the night before, he sent printed circulars to all members with a reminder that he would organize transport to the poll. On the night of the voting he hired conveyances to bring in members from all round the district. On their arrival at the hotel where the meeting was being held they found him waiting with treats of wine, whisky and beer. The offering of beer or other drinks is probably what Alfred Cox, for many years the Medical Secretary of the BMA, had in mind when in his influential *Among the Doctors* he says that 'many' lodge appointments were secured by 'bribery and corruption' (Cox, 1950, p. 57). However, the doctor who handed out drinks in this case lost the election to another colleague who 'just sent in' his application (*BMJ*, 23 January 1904, p. 197).

Moreover, there is very little evidence that handing out drinks or offering other inducements was typical. Indeed it would have been wholly out of character for the otherwise sober (many were total abstainers) members of the branches of the large affiliated orders to have behaved this way, as suggested, perhaps, by the fact that in the case cited the drinks on offer did not affect the outcome. No doubt there were exceptions, and no doubt some (perhaps many) of the local dividing societies functioned in this manner, but I can find no evidence that it was the norm, or even widespread.

Such conduct was also incompatible with the esteem in which doctors were held by the friendly societies, not to mention the self-esteem of most doctors. The medical officer was a highly respected society member; he would be given a place of honour at the annual dinner; certainly in after-dinner speeches lodge officers would generally sing the doctor's praises; after a few years of loyal service gifts of gold or silver would be presented; and on retirement he would be presented with valuable gifts for himself and his wife. Presentations on retirement had been the norm throughout the century. For example, members of the Lord Portman Lodge of Manchester Unity which met in Fleet Street, presented Dr Wilson with a silver tea pot on his retirement after twenty-three years. The chairman said the gift was a token of 'the very high appreciation' of members for his services and as an acknowledgement of their esteem for his 'unbounded kindness and gentlemanly bearing' toward them (*Monthly Review of Friendly Societies*, May 1865, p. 311).

Such banding together to appoint a branch medical officer had an additional advantage for the consumer, but also one disadvantage. The cost was that the individual enjoyed less choice. The majority decision determined who the doctor would be, and sometimes there was a minority that was more or less dissatisfied. The appointment of two or more medical officers to a society, however, went a great deal of the way towards solving this problem.

The early method of increasing professional incentives to defy their own cartels was to appoint a single medical officer to each society or branch. There was a second reason for favouring this device. Each society wanted to protect its sick fund from imposition, and the requirement that each member must obtain a certificate of sickness from the same doctor helped to ensure uniformity of treatment. A doctor who was too strict, or too lax, or inconsistent, could be dispensed with. This factor was undoubtedly the reason that many societies persisted with a single medical officer.

The appointment of one or more medical officers to a branch was not the only device used. The most notable alternative was the closed panel system under which doctors were placed on an approved list of doctors from which members could freely choose (see below, pp. 129, 158). This was not quite so attractive to doctors because it offered no guaranteed income, only the opportunity to compete with other doctors on the panel. But many doctors did join such schemes. For the consumer the attraction was that wider choice was available from among a list of doctors who had accepted the conditions laid down for inclusion on the panel. The conditions included prices, standards, and the range of services covered.

Rulebooks and Complaints: 'A Hundred Ignorant and Boorish Taskmasters'

There was little or no control of clinical judgement. And this was rarely at issue. Nor did it need to be, for if a society doubted a doctor's competence they could dispense with his services. The control was exercised through the rules of each society. These laid down the duties of the medical officer. Among the rules was provision for complaints to be made, usually for 'neglect' and 'delay'. Friendly society branches looked upon their medical officer as an official of the society, subject to the branch rules in the same way as any other member. Indeed, it was the custom in most societies for doctors to be required to become at least honorary members (BMA, CPR, 1905, p. 11). A procedure was laid down which enabled both sides to put their case, usually with an appeal available to the society's district level of organization.

Contrary to Titmuss' claim that doctors 'had no right of appeal under the "administrative law"' of the friendly societies (see above p. 71), doctors did enjoy a right of appeal when dissatisfied with lodge disciplinary procedures. A Foresters' court in Brierley Hill, for example, sacked its medical officer despite the non-attendance of the member who was complaining about him. The doctor took his case to the district organization, which upheld his appeal (*Lancet*, 1873, vol. 2, pp. 464–5).

And in most cases, very careful arrangements were made for both complaints and appeals. This also applied to the medical institutes. For example, the 1909 rules of the Luton Friendly Societies Medical Institute laid down the procedure for the arbitration of disputes. If a doctor or a member was not satisfied with the way the committee handled a complaint they could deposit 10s and have the dispute judged by a special committee of non-members drawn from the population of Luton. A panel of five non-members was maintained to hear disputes. When an appeal was lodged three of the five were chosen by lot to hear the case. Their decision was binding. And the vast majority of medical institutes had similar procedures.

The Norwich and Wolverhampton institutes, for example, both appointed official arbitrators (PRO MH77/93; PRO MH81/54). In 1934 the long-established procedure of the Norwich Friendly Societies Medical Institute provided for two levels of appeal against decisions of the committee. A member with a complaint against the doctors, the committee, or anyone else, brought it first to the management committee. If dissatisfied he could appeal to the arbitration committee of ten individuals appointed from among the delegates to the annual meeting. If the complaint was from a delegate's own branch, the delegate played no part in the arbitration committee proceedings. If dissatisfied with the decision, the member could appeal to the final arbitration committee, which comprised seven final arbitrators, four of whom were members of affiliated friendly societies but not officeholders or delegates, and three of whom were members of friendly societies not affiliated to the institute. Complaining members were allowed to be accompanied by up to two other members to assist them in putting their case (Norwich FSMI, *Rules*, 1934, rules 21–3 in PRO MH81/54).

We can get closest to an understanding of the relationship between doctors and lodges by examining surviving minute books. A representative case was the relationship between the medical officer and members of the Middlesbrough-based Court Erimus of the AOF (Court William Bryant until 1866). We can trace the relationship from the court's foundation in 1863 until 1948.

The original court surgeon, appointed in 1863, proved unsatisfactory and in June 1865 'in consequence of many complaints' received, he was replaced. The following January, probably as a result of a request from the new court surgeon, the annual fee per member was raised from 2s 6d to 3s 0d. In 1871 the much-respected Dr Simpson died. As with many doctors who were respected by society members, he had been a trustee of the court, responsible with two other trustees for investing court funds. He was replaced by Dr Park, who held office until 1878 when he resigned. He was also well respected, and after about eighteen months in office his annual fee was increased from 3s 0d to 4s 0d per member. He had served as an auditor of the court and appears to have attended court meetings. When he left, the court joined with a neighbouring court to present him with a testimonial for his 'kind and best attention' demonstrated over eight years.

The new medical officer was Dr Andson, but he was asked to accept a lower fee, and agreed to accept the position for 3s 6d. He had held office for ten years when, in 1888, a member brought a formal charge against him under the court rules for failing to visit when requested. The charge was made in writing according to the rules. Dr Andson was given a copy and given the prescribed fourteen days' notice to appear before the arbitration committee. At the meeting of the twelve-strong arbitration committee, the charge, made by one Bro. Smithson, was read aloud along with the relevant society rules. The minutes imply, without explicitly saying so, that Dr Andson had been drinking heavily before attending the meeting. He was asked to reply to the charge. He said he was surprised by it because he had been a friend of Bro. Smithson's. He then blamed his servants for failing to pass the message on to him. The court secretary reminded him that the statement which had just been read made the claim that Bro. Smithson's daughter had given the message to Dr Andson personally on two separate occasions. Dr Andson's resistance crumbled. The minutes then record that the doctor 'seemed to be in a state as he could not account for the neglect but he was willing to apologise to the member and also to promise to be more attentive to his duties' in the future. He was asked to retire from the room whilst the decision was made.

A number of members said it was wilful neglect and that they found his excuse very 'lame'. One commented that 'seeing the state he was in when attending the meeting' he was not a fit and proper person to be medical officer. Then a motion was put that Dr Andson should be required to (a) pay the bill given to Bro. Smithson by the other doctor he had had to call in; (b) pay the society the cost of calling the arbitration committee meeting; and that (c) he be censured. An amendment was moved that he should be required to pay only the other doctor's bill, but this was lost six to four, and the main proposition carried. Dr Andson told the committee that he agreed with the decision and asked for his apology to be conveyed to the whole court and to the member he had 'injured'. It only remained for the committee to consider whether to recommend the court to sack him. A motion to sack him was moved but lost. Leniency was decided upon. It was his first offence and it was resolved that, provided he 'reformed his conduct' he should retain office. At its next meeting in March the court upheld the decision of the arbitration committee. Dr Andson had a right of appeal to the district committee but did not exercise it.

However, it appears that Dr Andson did not mend his ways, and after having been allowed a few months' grace he was sacked by the June court meeting. The decision was not unanimous, but an attempt to reinstate him failed. At a special meeting nominations were called for his replacement. Drs Scanlan, Bateman, and Cook were nominated and a ballot taken. Dr Scanlan won by thirty votes to ten and five respectively.

Dr Scanlan accepted the post at 3s 6d per member per year, and seems to have proved very satisfactory to members. In April 1890 the court contemplated joining the medical institute which was being planned. They decided not to join (Ancient Order of Foresters, Court Erimus 4185, *Minute Book*, 1863–91). In May

1894 Dr Scanlan became a member of the branch and was presented with an 'elaborate framed emblem'. In December he became a trustee and sub-chief ranger (vice-chairman). In June 1895 he became chief ranger (chairman), a position which rotated annually. In May 1896 a special committee was appointed to consider his 'valuable service', and as a result, he was presented with a 9 carat gold past chief ranger's medal and badge, an honour not accorded to every past chief ranger. Until about 1901 he seems to have been a regular attender of meetings, but after this his attendances were less frequent (*Minute Book*, 1891–1901). By this time the court had about 330 male members, plus about 180 wives or widow members. This would have given Dr Scanlan an annual income of around £90. At the time some assistants embarked on their careers for an annual salary of less than this sum.

But Dr Scanlan was not immune from criticism. In December 1903 a member had written a letter to Dr Scanlan which the court found 'offensive', and which violated court rules. The court passed a vote of confidence in Dr Scanlan. In 1904 the court once again considered joining the medical institute, and again rejected the proposal. In July 1909 a complaint was received about Dr Scanlan. He was sent a copy and wrote to the court answering the charge. The dispute appears to have been over whether or not a member should have been recommended for the Forester's convalescent home in Bridlington. A member with tuberculosis had wanted to be sent there, but separate arrangements were made for TB sufferers and the court upheld Dr Scanlan's correct decision and wrote to him assuring him of their continued confidence. Dr Scanlan continued as medical officer on the same terms until he resigned on the eve of the National Insurance medical benefit scheme which began in January 1913.

At the last minute, however, he was asked to act for those members not covered by the National Insurance scheme and accepted, but at the much higher rate of 8s 6d per member, an increase of 5s 0d. The court again contemplated joining the medical institute, but once again decided to retain Dr Scanlan for members left out of the government scheme. He retained office, serving uninsured members and children until at least 1925 (*Minute Books*, 1902–13, 1913–26).

Consumer Choice After the 1911 Act

The pre-1911 disciplinary procedures were fair to doctor and patient alike and tended to maintain high standards of care. Competition and society rules also tended to widen the range of special services covered by contract practice. The view that consumers were too ignorant to be allowed to exercise such power is not supported by the evidence so far presented.

Ironically, these devices were dismantled for the insured population in 1911 as a result of professional propaganda using as its slogan 'free choice of doctor', implying that such choice meant competition and consequent consumer power. As I will show, doctors openly intended, and in practice obtained, the very opposite outcome.

Among the unfavourable judgements made on contract practice was the contention that there was no free choice of doctor. This was an argument used to good effect by the doctors in their 1911 propaganda. And according to Braithwaite, it proved a very influential argument. The doctors, he said, 'had the whole House on the run with this specious cry of "free choice of doctor"' (Bunbury, 1957, p. 198). Certainly, Lloyd George had swallowed the argument. He helped to confuse the issue, by asserting that he had always been in favour of free choice, commenting that, 'No man who could afford to do otherwise would have a doctor prescribed for him by any club or society' (Hansard, 1 August 1911, col. 318).

That the Act widened freedom of choice has also been accepted without qualification by recent scholars. Among the various systems of contract practice, Gilbert found the friendly societies to be 'unquestionably' the best. But he criticizes contract practice for contradicting 'the essential tenet of medical ethics', mutual choice by patient and healer: 'Friendly society practice was contract practice; the doctor was an employee of the society. His patients did not choose him; nor could he refuse service to any of them' (1966, p. 309).

The 1911 National Insurance Act is widely held to have given the beneficiaries of the Act freedom of choice, when hitherto they had none. Was this true? Were club members denied freedom of choice among medical practitioners? The first thing to understand is that there were a wide variety of arrangements for health care available among the friendly societies. The most common was the lodge system. Each branch employed a single medical officer. We have already considered how this system enhanced the consumer's power in the marketplace. By the turn of the century solo lodge practice was tending to develop into an approved panel system, as more members demanded wider choice of doctor. In some localities there had long been choice. Under the 1840 rules of the Sheffield District, for example, any member of the twenty-plus lodges in Sheffield could choose any of the other lodge surgeons within the district. There was also a deputizing scheme. From 1837 every surgeon in the district was required to deputize for other surgeons who were unable to respond to requests for a visit because they were not at home (Siddall, 1924, p. 10). By the turn of the century a variety of arrangements offering choice existed as the BMA's own contract practice report shows (e.g. BMA, CPR, 1905, Appendix D; Brabrook, 1898, p. 71).

In around 1876 in Leicester the friendly societies had separated medical attendance from dispensing. They had tried to do the dispensing through local chemists but had replaced that arrangement with their own dispensary. It supplied not only medicines, but also cod liver oil, dressings and nutritional items not normally supplied by doctors. By 1911 they had in addition a board of thirty-two surgeons who would attend and prescribe for all members. Members could choose freely among them (*Oddfellows Magazine*, July 1911, pp. 353–4).

In 1910 a scheme was under way to extend choice among doctors in the North London District of Manchester Unity. This permitted transfer by right to any lodge doctor in the area who had agreed to enter the scheme. About 80 per cent of lodge surgeons had agreed to participate (*Oddfellows Magazine*, February 1911, pp. 70–1). By 1910 it was common for members to pay their sick pay contributions into one lodge and their 'medical pence' into another. One newly-opened lodge very rapidly had fifty such contributors (*Oddfellows Magazine*, September 1910, p. 664). In some cases payment to the lodge surgeon was compulsory, but by the 1880s this was exceptional in Manchester Unity (*Oddfellows Magazine*, April 1886, pp. 104–5). About 30 per cent of members in the North London District of Manchester Unity were not paying medical contributions into their own lodge. Many would have been paying the surgeons of other lodges (*Oddfellows Magazine*, December 1910, p. 897). A lodge secretary, also probably from London, told the *Oddfellows Magazine* that 150 of his 600 members did not pay their medical contribution to him. He thought about half paid into other lodges and that the others could have done so if they wished. Surgeons were allowed to refuse them but over many years it was his experience that they rarely did so. He knew of only one such case out of 'scores' of others (*Oddfellows Magazine*, December 1910, p. 897).

There was also provision for those lodge members who moved to a new locality. They were known as distant members and could secure the services of the local lodge surgeon – though some surgeons did have the right to refuse, depending on local custom (*Oddfellows Magazine*, January 1886, pp. 22–5). In some districts it had also long been the practice to provide for 'travelling' members. Under the 1840 rules of the Sheffield District of Manchester Unity the surgeons were required to attend without additional charge members from other lodges travelling in search of work (Siddall, 1924, p. 10). Before the 1911 Act the local dividing societies were also making arrangements for their distant members. In 1908 and 1909 the National Federation of Dividing Societies was organizing improved medical care for their members who lived at an inconvenient distance from their own society's doctor. Members could pay 1s 1d per quarter by post and secure attendance from any one of a hundred doctors on an approved list. Families would be attended for a further 1s 1d (*BMJ*, 13 February 1909, p. 425).

As we have seen, in the largest of the affiliated orders, Manchester Unity, there was already considerable freedom of choice. And new schemes were emerging to increase choice, where it was wanted. The situation was not the same in the Ancient Order of Foresters, the second largest of the affiliated orders. The medical contribution was compulsory for those living within a stated distance of the branch meeting place (usually three miles) (RCPL, Appendix VII, Qs 77385–6). Apart from the desire to regulate sick pay claims, this was also because it was felt to be an unreasonable imposition on the doctors not to require payment from every local member. Doctors provided services for the whole society as well as for individuals. Most AOF branches had a single medical officer, but several branches had more than one, and some had five or six medical officers, with the right of choice between them at quarterly or six-monthly intervals (RCPL, 1909, Appendix VII, Qs 77322, 77475).

But the compulsory contribution rule could be, and was, evaded. Rule 41 in the 1907 rulebook provided for all those members who lived more than three miles from their branch meeting place to enjoy the services of any other court medical officer for the same contribution. (A similar rule had long existed (see AOF, *General Laws*, 1857).) It was common practice for men to join a branch near their place of work, not near their residence, and so many members had effective free choice. And as public transport improved around the turn of the century, it became very common for men to live well away from their place of work. It was certainly not necessary for a member who did not like his branch medical officer to just put up with him, as some branch by-laws explicitly laid down. The rules of Guisborough's Court Old Abbey, for example, laid down that 'any member who thinks [it] proper to employ any other than the Surgeon of this Court is at liberty to do so' (AOF, Court Old Abbey 603, *Rules*, 1877, rule 37). Some members of the AOF opted out altogether, but the permanent secretary estimated in 1907 that 95 per cent of its 700,000 members contributed for medical care (RCPL, 1909, Appendix VII, Q. 77480).

In addition to the alternative schemes available members were naturally free to consult other doctors for a fee. Families would often have more than one doctor: one for the man, one for the wife, and one for the children (*Lancet*, 1896, vol. 2, p. 597). One doctor who had served a Foresters' court for nineteen years reported that about thirty of his 162 adult members called in other doctors when they were sick. Many members also called in other doctors when their wives or children were ill. They thought it 'better form'. It gave them 'tone' (BMA, CPR, p. 39).

The second type of health cover provided by the friendly societies was the approved panel system. Consumers appointed doctors to a panel from which members could choose. Membership of the panel depended on conformity with conditions laid down by consumers, particularly with agreed fees. Over the years there had been experimentation with such systems, some based on capitation fee payment and some not.

Some friendly societies developed ticket systems. In the 1860s the ticket systems were in their infancy. In a part of Hampshire, for instance, members of one scheme paid 4s per year. Each member had a supply of tickets and doctors were refunded the cash value of the tickets handed them by members. A home visit was worth 2s, a surgery consultation cost 1s 6d, and medicine without consultation cost a 9d ticket. There were additional payments for accidents and operations (*BMJ*, 23 October 1869, p. 457). Deposit friendly societies commonly used a ticket system, dividing the cost between the common fund and the member's own account (see *Lancet*, 1871, vol. 2, pp. 790–1). This system was developed on a large scale by the National Deposit Friendly Society. It paid its doctors 2s 6d for a home visit, inclusive of medicines, and 1s 6d per surgery consultation (*BMJ*, 18 January 1896, p. 172). In 1911 the NDFS had over 300,000 members.

In some localities societies experimented with a 'medical pool'. In one society contributions were paid to the lodge, and two doctors saw members as private patients at ordinary fees. The fees were paid by the lodge from the common fund. In the first year (1882) the scheme cost £32 with 160 members; in 1883, £37 with 161 members; in 1884, £59 with 166 members; and in 1885, £82 with 172 members. The scheme had to be abandoned as too costly and contract practice was reinstated (*Oddfellows Magazine*, July 1890, p. 219). Such schemes were attempted frequently but were often abandoned. This was chiefly because they tended to be too expensive. Separate payment for every visit cost a good deal more than members could afford.

The third type of cover offered by the friendly societies was the medical institute, which employed one or more full-time medical officers. Usually there was more than one doctor, and so members could choose between them, although obviously, if there was only one, members had no choice.

During the doctors' campaign to amend the National Insurance Bill they sometimes cleverly appealed to the disgruntled minority which could be left by majority voting. But dissatisfied friendly society members were few. First, this was because a disgruntled minority did not have to remain so in perpetuity. There was the possibility of overturning the decision at regular intervals. Most appointments were for fixed terms of three or six months. But more than this, the individual could always resign and join a different society or branch. Abiding by the majority decision is not very onerous in a voluntary association which one can easily quit. Members are self-selected in the first place. This is quite different from the situation in a compulsory association like a nation state or a closed shop.

Moreover, the free choice espoused by the doctors was not in very big demand. The BMA had been pressing its policy of guaranteed access to contract practice for any willing doctor for some years by 1911, but it had not been widely accepted because it was not wanted. The reason was that the appointment of a single lodge medical officer (or for that matter, the appointment of any *limited* number of medical officers) facilitated control of the doctor's conduct. This was wanted by the friendly societies for two reasons: (a) to retain control of their funds; and (b) to maintain the standard of medical care. Their power was the result of banding together; to abandon their unity was to put themselves singly at the mercy of an organized producer group. Some modern intellectuals (e.g. Gilbert, 1966; Klein, 1973) disapprove of the friendly societies for attempting to protect their funds. To the modern intellectual, reared amidst the apparent superabundance of the welfare state financed by the ever pliant taxpayer, protecting the funds seems a bit mean. But to take this view is to misunderstand how friendly society members thought. Because members were part of a voluntary association they had a keen sense that the funds were their own money. For the friendly society member, to impose on the funds was simply to impose on other people with little to call their own. To protect the funds against such imposition seemed to them to require no further justification.

To sum up: before the 1911 Act there was, therefore, a degree of choice and where wider choice was wanted it was being provided. But at any particular moment, there were minorities in friendly society branches who would have preferred a different doctor. The Act gave them free choice among panel practitioners.

When the Act was passed most society members kept their previous doctor. And, ironically, for some friendly society members the Act brought a loss of choice. From January 1913 until April 1920 it was possible to change doctors only annually; and from 1920 until 1924, only half-yearly in June and

December if six months' notice had been given. Friendly societies which allowed members to change, often permitted changes to be made at quarterly intervals. (From 1924 insured persons not connected with a medical institute could change at any time, though this was later changed to quarterly intervals.) Moreover, the freedom of choice of the person insured under the Act was deliberately limited to a choice between individual medical practitioners. The other two arrangements possible under the Act under section 15(3) and section 15(4) (see pp. 160ff) were severely curtailed.

But the fact that there was or was not choice in the sense in which the BMA used the term is not the real issue. What mattered was whether or not the consumer had the power to alter the conduct of doctors – either directly or indirectly – in the interests of patients. Free choice is normally valued because it is held to give the patient influence over the doctor. But if the patients are all isolated and the professionals tightly organized this is not necessarily the result.

The BMA's Explicit Plans to Stamp Out Competition

There is no doubt from the medical journals that the BMA was seeking to stamp out competition. It used a variety of devices, but the two main methods were: (a) mis-using the power of the GMC to ban conduct which helped the consumer to differentiate between doctors, such as canvassing and advertising; and (b) the establishment of cartels to fix rates of pay and conditions to which *every* practitioner would adhere.

One method by which they sought to enforce uniform rates and conditions and thus eliminate competition was to discourage the appointment of a single medical officer to each friendly society branch. The device used was to press for members to be given 'free choice' among all the practitioners of a district. The reasoning is made explicit in the report of the medico-political committee in 1905. The attractions of acquiring a large number of patients at once through a club appointment encouraged competition: 'In the competition between medical practitioners the prospect of obtaining an entire club appears sometimes to induce practitioners to descend to unworthy practices of which they would not otherwise be guilty.' The remedy was for contract practice to be open to all doctors who wished to participate. This, the report contended, was good for both doctor and patient. The patient had 'choice', and the doctor achieved 'independence'; and the arrangement was 'good for the profession as a whole' because it did away with the 'abuse due to competition' (BMA, CPR, 1905, p. 6). These abuses were canvassing and advertising.

Opinions among doctors submitting evidence to the inquiry of 1905 were divided, but a large number felt that contract practice was 'absolutely necessary', and the medico-political committee felt it was 'inevitable' that contract practice should be retained in at least some areas. Contract practice had, according to the BMA, three attractions: (a) certainty of income, including the avoidance of bad debts; (b) it served as an introduction to families; and (c) if one doctor did not take contract patients others would. In the BMA's view, only the avoidance of bad debts was a valid reason for favouring contract practice. The other reasons could all be removed by eliminating competition (BMA, CPR, 1905, p. 9). The BMA inquiry found that the system of dividing work among all the practitioners in a district had grown more common, and 211 cases were reported to them. But overall, instances of the system were 'relatively very infrequent' (BMA, CPR, pp. 6, 10).

Similar arguments had been advanced in connection with the National Deposit Friendly Society system, a scheme favoured by many doctors. National Deposit members paid flat-rate annual contributions which entitled them to claim from the society a fixed proportion (usually two thirds or three quarters) of doctors' fees. In 1904 the BMA's medico-political committee had investigated the scheme and recommended that no such system should be allowed to develop. They disliked it because it tended to lower fees. This was because doctors serving National Deposit members tended to become an approved panel of practitioners, who conformed to fees fixed by consumers. In each district the NDFS was said to 'distinguish between those medical practitioners who have indicated willingness to accept the scale of charges and those who do not'. And representatives of the society often called on doctors to encourage them to accept work on the society's terms. As a result society members tended to employ approved practitioners 'to the exclusion of their neighbours, and thus underselling is brought about' (*BMJ* Supplement, 28 May 1904, pp. 132–3; BMA, CPR, 1905, p. 26).

Thus the 'choice' offered to the consumer by the 1911 Act was explicitly at the expense of power over the profession. The prospect of winning a single patient here and there was not sufficient inducement to doctors to defy their colleagues. The prospect of winning a couple of hundred or so was. Free choice sounded good, but it was the choice of the atomized consumer from among the members of a producer cartel, who supplied similar services on similar terms, so that the choice was between *identical* and not different suppliers. The essence of competition is that it facilitates *comparison* between *different* suppliers.

Control in Panel Practice and the NHS
In 1911 most of the organizations representing medical consumers had been stripped of their direct responsibility for the provision of primary medical care. But the medical institutes remained, and those approved societies which had formerly offered medical benefit retained an interest in, if no power over, medical provision under the 1911 Act. In 1948 these organizations were either dissolved or swept aside. Direct representation of insured persons also disappeared. Three fifths of the members of the former insurance committees had been direct representatives of the insured population, appointed by approved societies. The new executive councils not only had more professional members, their lay membership was nominated by local authorities. As Professor Titmuss conceded in 1959, the working classes may have benefited from the NHS, but the middle classes 'benefited even more, and the medical profession most of all' (p. 318).

The general practitioner service under the NHS was organized on very similar lines to inter-war panel practice. The local insurance committees were simply replaced by local executive councils, bodies with very similar powers. There was one major difference: professional representation was dramatically increased. The insurance committees had been made up as follows: three fifths of the members were elected by insured persons; one fifth by the local authority; and of the remaining fifth, two were elected by the medical profession, one was a doctor appointed by the local authority, and the remainder were appointed by the Ministry of Health.

The executive councils were half-professional, half-lay bodies, with two thirds of the lay members appointed by the local authority and one third by the minister. There were twenty-four members plus the chairman, who was appointed by the local authority. Of the twelve lay members, eight were appointed by the local authority and four by the minister. Of the twelve professionals, seven were appointed by the local medical committee, three by the local dental committee, and two by the local pharmaceutical committee (Ross, 1952, p. 108).

These gains were consolidated by the 1974 reforms. The Family Practitioner Committees have thirty members appointed as follows: eleven by the Area Health Authority; four by the local authority; eight by the local medical committee (one of whom must be an opthalmic medical practitioner); three by the local dental committee; two by the local pharmaceutical committee; two by the local optical committee (one of whom must be an opthalmic optician and the other a dispensing optician). Professional power continued unscathed through the 1982 reforms, and there is no sign that the present government will do much to redress the balance.

Joint selection and approved panels were techniques for putting doctors under pressure to meet consumer wants. Unsatisfactory doctors were filtered out, and doctors who wished to avoid this fate found it necessary to adjust their conduct accordingly. In addition to these methods, which in the end rested on the blunt instrument of dismissal, the friendly societies also evolved procedures for checking the conduct of doctors in post. Their complaints procedures made it possible to keep doctors on their toes when their conduct fell below the standard desired by consumers but was not bad enough to warrant dismissal. I have already described the complaints procedure of the friendly societies. I turn now to a comparison between the societies' procedure and the government complaints machinery established under the 1911 Act.

As Professor Klein has argued, the 1911 Act 'marked a giant step forward in the emancipation of the medical profession from lay control'. The complaints machinery introduced in 1911, which remains essentially the same today, was introduced 'not as an attempt to fortify the position of the consumer but as a salvage operation designed to save something from the wreck of lay control over medical services'. The 1911 deal represents 'the first rung in the ladder leading to the syndicalist system of professional control over the health services' (Klein, 1973, p. 60).

Klein concedes that the friendly societies secured lay involvement in the disciplinary machinery set up under the 1911 scheme, but he can not quite bring himself to give them any credit for this. They were not 'fighting for the idea of lay participation as such', rather they were trying to protect their funds against doctors who might be too lavish in issuing sick certificates. They were protecting 'not their principles but their pockets' (1973, p. 66). This interpretation is, I believe, undeservedly hard on the friendly societies, whose commitment to self-government as a matter of principle was second to none.

Klein cites the records of complaints made between 1920 and 1924 in support of his thesis that: 'On balance the Approved Societies do not seem to have been concerned to develop the potentialities of the system for ensuring a better service to the consumer, but to limit the risks to those paying out insurance and to enforce a contract as strictly as possible' (1973, p. 72). He draws this conclusion even though for every one complaint about irregular certification there were two others about poor service, such as non-visiting, inadequate treatment, and unjustified charging of fees (ibid., p. 70). Klein's complaint is that the approved societies were concerned with 'preventing the abuse of public funds' rather than with improving the quality of medical care (ibid., p. 73).

Another of the costs of the NHS identified by Professor Klein is that when the approved societies disappeared in 1948 the balance of power between professional and consumer in the complaints machinery shifted in favour of the professional. The rules provided for patients to be represented by their approved society and for the doctor to be represented by the local medical committee. When the approved societies were dissolved the patient had no organizational backing, while the doctors retained theirs (ibid., p. 69).

The friendly society tradition was based on the rules of natural justice. There are two main principles: *audi alteram partem*, 'hear the other side'; and *nemo judex in causa sua*, 'no man may be a judge in his own cause'. Underlying this philosophy was the belief that both sides had an equal right to have their case heard and that essential to the process was the independence of those judging the issue. Their rules therefore provided for the appointment of arbitration committees comprised of individuals with no axe to grind.

The view of the doctors was the opposite. No one should judge professional conduct except the professional, the professional should be judged only by his peers. Doctors have often asserted that this notion is in the public interest, but without exception it has been accompanied by an ethic of professional loyalty which strongly frowned upon criticism of one's fellows. And as the Merrison committee (1975, p. 82) found, the ethic of 'unthinking loyalty' is today as strong as ever.

Under the NHS the complaints machinery is essentially the same as when it was introduced in 1913. Since 1974 a panel made up of three doctors and three lay persons with a mutually accepted chairman considers complaints. But the whole procedure is limited in scope. The question being asked, according to Professor Klein, is: 'whether the doctor has carried out the duties for which he is being paid, not whether he is a competent practitioner' (1983, p. 162). It provides little protection for the consumer, as Klein's (1973) study shows.

Conclusion

In the marketplace devices serving to increase consumer power at the expense of the organized profession emerged, as did mechanisms functioning as information-supplying devices to help overcome the consumer's relative lack of knowledge. These were dismantled by the state at the behest of the doctors. As a means of protecting the consumer from either professional power or superior professional knowledge, the state subsequently proved to be far less effective than did the consumer's own spontaneous organizations for self protection.

8
National Insurance Medical Benefit: Still Second Class?

In Chapter 4 I considered the problem of consumer ignorance. In particular I examined the claim that consumer dominance produced results harmful for doctor and patient alike. In this Chapter I will consider what improvements in the standard of service the 1911 Act brought.

One of the criticisms of contract practice was that it provided a lower standard of service than that offered to private patients. But complaints about the standard of medical care did not end with the 1911 National Insurance Act. There were complaints that patients were referred to hospitals whenever their case became demanding; that doctors were reluctant to make home visits; that doctors took too many patients for efficient service; that private patients received priority over panel patients; and the argument continued about whether or not minor surgery was covered by the capitation fee (*Oddfellows Magazine*, December 1921, pp. 586–9; *Foresters Miscellany*, October 1923, p. 588; and *Foresters Miscellany*, November 1923, p. 601).

In 1945 there were still complaints that private practice was superior. Labour's manifesto insisted that money should 'no longer be the passport to the best treatment'. And as late as 1946 complaints were being voiced by doctors that panel practice had undesirable effects on the doctor–patient relationship. The patient called on the doctor for trivial reasons, and there was a general loss of mutual respect, with the patient taking the view, 'I am entitled to it and I am going to have it' (*BMJ*, Supplement, 17 August 1946, pp. 63–4).

In 1923 the coroner of North London made a strong attack on the panel system: 'It put a premium on scamped work and inefficiency.' The worst work, he thought, was being done by the men drawing the largest incomes. The panel system was 'a miserable failure' (*Oddfellows Magazine*, July 1923, p. 495). The coroner's criticism was denounced by the BMA as 'an unwarrantable attack' on panel practitioners (*Oddfellows Magazine*, July 1923, p. 496).

In 1924 the secretary of the NCFS said there were 'ample' grounds for complaint about panel doctors. A better system of certification was required, along with 'the total abolition of queues outside surgeries, the degradation of the differentiation between panel and private services, the swollen number of people on doctors' panels' (*Foresters Miscellany*, November 1923, pp. 615–16).

In the 1930s PEP (now the Policy Studies Institute) thought that panel practice in 'working-class areas' was not 'as efficient as it might be under different circumstances':

The panel doctor, at any rate in large towns, often has neither the facilities nor the equipment which, as precise diagnosis becomes daily more possible, are necessary to provide an adequate service. As a result he passes on his patients to the hospital and specialized clinics and often enough he tends to become little more than an agent for signing certificates. These tendencies are strengthened where, owing to the low remuneration he receives or the circumstances of the area in which he lives, the practitioner is forced to undertake more work than he can conscientiously perform. The panel doctor's difficulties are often further accentuated by the lack of clerical assistance and by the difficulty of obtaining laboratory services.

Personal contact between the panel doctor and his patients is also often lost since the doctor and his family, fearing the social isolation of the poor urban area, live in more congenial surroundings while the doctor's work is done from a lock-up surgery (PEP, 1937, p. 162).

The Panel Doctor

During the early months of medical benefit some doctors appear to have intimated to patients that their treatment would improve if an additional fee was paid. As a result the National Insurance Amending Act of 1913 included a provision prohibiting doctors from accepting any fee for treating panel patients (Gilbert, 1966, p. 441). This did not stop the practice. In that year, for example, it was reported to the West Sussex Insurance Committee that a doctor had informed a panel patient that he could not give the patient as good a service as he used to give when the patient had been treated privately. The insurance committee very strongly criticized the doctor (*National Insurance Gazette*, 20 September 1913, p. 616). The Ministry of Health reported to the Royal Commission that a 'considerable number of cases have occurred in which the irregular charging of fees by practitioners has necessitated disciplinary action,' although the Ministry felt the practice was decreasing (RCNHI, 1926, Appendices, p. 86).

In giving evidence to the Royal Commission, the president and secretary of the National Conference of Friendly Societies raised no complaints about the medical service, but the vice-president said he thought from his own direct experience that it left 'much to be desired'. There was no question in his mind 'but that there is still today a distinction made between the panel patient and the private patient'. There was a distinction made 'in the treatment and in the respect generally' paid to insured and private patients (RCNHI, 1926, Qs 11003–011). The Royal Commission, however, rejected the view that doctors gave an inferior service to panel patients compared with private patients (RCNHI, *Report*, pp. 37–8).

The Honorary Secretary of the Joint Committee of Approved Societies gave evidence that panel practice offered an inferior service. 'Miserable petty surcharges' had been imposed on doctors for prescribing a five-grain pill when a three- or four-grain pill would have sufficed. Such decisions would have been unchallenged when dealing with a private patient. 'It was a sin,' he commented, 'for a flavouring essence to be put into an insured person's medicine.' And at one time the insured patient's bandages 'were to be drab and grey', not white as in the case of the private patient. Such attitudes applied particularly to London. In one respect National Insurance had made matters worse than under voluntary contract practice. A panel doctor had to take into account 'whether his attainments were within the professional competence of his professional brethren.' In earlier days if a doctor had the ability 'he exercised it' (RCNHI, 1926, Qs 8029–31, 8091–7). This was a reference to the terms of service of the panel doctor, which laid down that 'all proper and necessary medical services other than those involving the application of special skill and experience of a degree or kind which general practitioners as a class cannot reasonably be expected to possess' must be provided. This was not the rule applied in club practice. If a doctor had a skill he used it. There was no levelling down to the average. And this remained the case in the medical institutes. The 1934 rules of the Norwich FSMI, for example, required medical officers to 'prescribe and give the best medical treatment in their power to all sick patients' (Rule 20 in PRO MH81/54).

One of the criticisms of contract practice was that doctors had a financial incentive to offer a low standard of service. Lloyd George had made much of this. He had contended that the friendly societies would 'utilize their influence to depress the standard of medical attendance to save themselves.' It was not, he argued, 'in the interests of public health that you should have a body of 6,000,000 men in this country the interests of whose organization is rather to restrict the development of medical attendance.'

He went on to identify three differences between the new and old arrangements. Drugs, he argued, would be 'for the first time' supplied. There would be free choice of doctor. And, the friendly societies would benefit by transferring their costs to the public purse (Hansard, 1 August 1911, cols. 319–20). I have already referred to the freedom of choice issue. And very few friendly societies had been attracted by Lloyd George's argument that they would be better off without having to administer medical benefit.

His reference to drugs presumably meant that they would be supplied separately. But this was already done in Scotland and was the practice of the hundred or so medical institutes which Lloyd George had only reluctantly permitted to enter the scheme. But much more to the point, the government deliberately built into the scheme an arrangement intended to restrict doctors' freedom to prescribe (Eder, 1982, pp. 260–78). And when their early measures to control 'excessive prescribing' were deemed to have failed, additional measures were implemented in 1916.

The General Medical Benefit Fund, out of which all medical and drug expenses were to be paid, was divided into three smaller funds: the Panel Services Fund, the Institutions Fund, and the Special Arrangements Fund. The Panel Services Fund was the main fund, and was also divided into three. The Panel Fund was used to pay the doctors for their attendance, mainly according to the capitation rate. The Drug Fund paid for medicines, and the Drug Suspense Fund (sometimes called the 'floating sixpence') could be used for either medical attendance or drugs.

If the cost of drugs in the insurance committee area exceeded 1s 6d per head, but not the 2s 0d allocated, the difference between 2s 0d and the actual cost over 1s 6d went to the Panel Fund and thence to the doctors. If expenditure exceeded the 2s, the accounts of all chemists were scaled down so that the average came to 2s (RCNHI, 1926, Appendices, Ministry of Health, Appendix C, paras. 112–114).

Under this system, according to the Ministry of Health, 'doctors themselves had a financial interest in securing economy in prescribing.' From 1916, however, this device alone was not relied upon. A drug tariff was introduced along with other checks. Doctors in the form of the Panel Committees were required to investigate prescribing themselves. It was open to the insurance committees to impose a surcharge on a doctor for 'excessive prescribing'. This arrangement lasted until 1923. (The arrangement under which the practitioner 'had a speculative interest' in the floating sixpence had been abolished from January 1920.)

By the 1930s insurance committees in England and Wales were grouped into fifteen areas, each with a pricing bureau. Costs well above the average cost per insured person in the area could lead to a doctor being required to explain his reasons. He could be warned or the matter referred to the panel committee for disciplinary action. The Ministry of Health considered that there was still excessive prescribing in the 1930s (Annual Report of the Chief Medical Officer of the Ministry of Health, 1935 in PEP, 1937, p. 147).

However, the measures seem to have made a difference to prescribing habits in some areas, to the detriment of patients. According to the Ministry of Health in 1924 the arrangements then introduced to control prescribing had proved ineffective in many cases, whilst in some areas the measures had created the impression 'in the minds of certain doctors that expensive medicines were not available for their insured patients' (RCNHI, 1926, Appendices, Ministry of Health, Appendix C, para. 91). The Scottish Board of Health, however, had found that the doctors' 'financial interest in the "floating sixpence" was not, in itself, sufficient to control excessive and extravagant prescribing' (RCNHI, 1926, Appendices, Scottish Board of Health, Appendix C, para. 18).

The National Medical Union complained that London practitioners were under a definite disincentive not to prescribe freely. The fear of being investigated for excessive prescribing (understood as exceeding the average for the area) deterred doctors from prescribing as they normally would (RCNHI, 1926, Qs 15 882–92). For example, in 1918 the panel committee of the Croydon Insurance Committee found that the cost of drugs prescribed by a particular doctor 'was in excess of what was reasonably necessary for the adequate treatment of his insured persons, and that he prescribed on a scale and in a manner that is extravagant when judged by the standards of his colleagues.' It was felt that the doctor prescribed too many pills at once, included too many ingredients in his prescriptions, and used flavourings to excess. His drug bill was £29 compared with an average of £17 for six other doctors with a similar number of patients. The panel committee recommended that he be surcharged the difference of £12.

The proposal to surcharge the doctor met initial resistance. A councillor reminded the committee that under the 'floating sixpence' system doctors gained financially by cutting down on their prescriptions. He was not therefore surprised at the 'keen interest' shown by the panel committee in the matter (*Foresters Miscellany*, September 1918, pp. 434–5). Nevertheless, a surcharge was imposed on this and at least one other occasion.

In Coventry one doctor gave evidence that doctors had been exhorted by colleagues not to exceed a stated level of expenditure. Those that exceeded it were accused of 'not doing their best to earn the 6d for the whole lot' (RCNHI, 1926, Q. 16 610).

The Scottish Medical Guild complained that the National Insurance scheme had encouraged chemists 'to buy a cheap class of drug' (RCNHI, 1926, Qs 16 019–20; Appendices, Appendix L). In 1923 a member of the Medical Guild, also an Edinburgh employer, had complained that many of his employees got their prescriptions made up by non-panel chemists and paid a higher fee (*Foresters Miscellany*, March 1923, p. 135). This claim could be consistent with the evidence of the Retail Pharmacists Union, which complained that up to 1916 many chemists had lost money. They had had no control over prescribing, but the total expenditure was confined to 2s per head. Under this pressure it is possible that some chemists may have succumbed to temptation. But when questioned the RPU denied that inferior medicines were supplied to panel patients (Qs 18 066–77). That panel patients were given inferior treatment was also denied by the General Council of Panel Chemists (Scotland) (Appendices, Appendix LXIX, para. 6). On the other hand the Incorporated Society of Pharmacy and Drug Store Proprietors claimed there were cases of 'alteration of prescriptions by dispensing chemists for their own pecuniary benefit,' and cases of 'supplying short measure, inaccurate dispensing, and inferior articles' (Appendices, Appendix LXVI, para. 13; Qs 12 284–87).

In the days of contract practice there were complaints that because the doctor was paid a flat rate he had an incentive to prescribe cheap (and useless) medicines. Lloyd George, for instance, claimed that, 'In many cases drugs of the most expensive character were not supplied when they might have been' (Hansard, 1 August 1911, col. 318). As a result he favoured the separation of funding for drugs from funding for attendance.

Contract practice did put a ceiling on expenditure on drugs which may or may not have influenced the conduct of doctors. But, especially for the poor, it was a very considerable improvement on what had gone before. A Dr McCreadie told a meeting of AOF officers in Leith that the friendly society member experienced:

no fear of a heavy doctor's bill to hamper and hinder convalescence. There was no hesitation in taking the medicine provided as the sick brother had already paid for its supply. On the other hand, in his daily work among the working classes of Leith he had seen the house gradually emptied of everything that would sell. He had seen illness prolonged for want of necessary medical comforts and treatment; the visits of the physician dreaded on account of the difficulty to pay afterwards; the prescriptions lying unheeded owing to the lack of money to pay the chemist (*Foresters Miscellany*, August 1913, p. 288).

Under the 1911 Act there was still a limit on the amount that could be spent on medicines. Indeed, the scheme had deliberately built into it (until 1920) an incentive to doctors of exactly the same kind. Pressure to constrain prescribing continued throughout the scheme. The one arrangement which suffered from no such pressure, and which even its worst critics did not accuse of supplying insufficient or unsatisfactory medicines, the medical institute, was prohibited from expanding after 1911.

It was not until January 1938 that an agreement with the chemists which guaranteed them full payment for the medicine supplied came into effect. The annual report of the Ministry of Health commented that it had been 'felt for some time' that agreements which did not guarantee the chemist full payment for medicines supplied 'were not satisfactory' (MOH, *Annual Report*, 1938, p. 141).

The evidence does not enable a hard and fast conclusion to be drawn about the standard of prescribing after the 1911 Act. A definite sum of 1s 6d was earmarked for medicine. This formally eliminated the possibility that doctors might spend the capitation fee on themselves instead of on medicine. But before 1911 competitive pressures had been such that doctors could not get away with neglecting patients. Lloyd George claimed that the 1s 6d per patient per year allocated for drugs was an increase over pre-1911 levels (Hansard, Commons, 1914, vol. 59, cols. 670–71). Yet complaints were still regularly voiced that panel patients were not given the best. It is impossible to establish with absolute certainty the extent to which inferior or insufficient medicine was supplied either before or after 1911. But, one thing is clear: the volume of complaint does not seem to have abated after 1911. In the eyes of the consumer, at least, the paternalistic state appeared to have made no difference.

Other criticisms also continued to be voiced after the passing of the Act. Before 1911 the work of the GP was 'carried on under conditions of isolation from his professional colleagues to a greater extent perhaps than almost any other branch of the profession'. He lacked facilities for the exchange of ideas and for cooperation, thus cutting him off from 'ready access to new ideas at a time of rapid development of medical science' and depriving him of the benefit of professional criticism: 'The inevitable result . . . was that only exceptional individuals, having the intellectual and moral qualities necessary for efficient self-criticism, could escape the danger of a constant sagging down of technical efficiency' (MOH, 1919–20, p. 188).

The report of the chief medical officer went on to concede that by 1920 this problem had not been removed. This was blamed on the war. The standard of the medical service compared with the pre-1911 service was appraised as follows:

so far as the capabilities of the Insurance practitioners are concerned, the quality of the service given under the Insurance Acts is to be regarded as practically the same as that given by general practitioners to persons of the same economic position before and since the Act of 1911 came into operation. . .

This conclusion was subject only to any improvement that may have resulted from the pressure of administrative authorities and to improvements consequent upon the better pay of the doctors (MOH, 1919–20, p. 189).

Complaints about the isolation of GPs did not end in 1920. They were still being voiced in the 1930s, and are still heard today. The Royal Commission on the NHS of 1979 identified three main reasons for low standards in the GP service. The third of these was that GPs were 'often isolated and lack the close contact with professional colleagues which is available to those who work in hospitals'. The spread of health centres was thought to provide part of the answer (RCNHS, 1979, pp. 81–2).

Ironically, as we have seen, the medical institutes did bring doctors together, but their expansion was halted by the 1911 Act. The institutes also facilitated cooperation between doctors and chemists as the FSMA argued in 1946, but this argument was given short shrift by the Ministry.

A further complaint made about contract practice was that doctors would leave the contract work to their assistants. The 1911 Act did not change the situation. Alfred Cox, Medical Secretary of the BMA, gave evidence to the Royal Commission that the employment of assistants was unavoidable (RCNHI, 1926, Q. 14739). And complaints that assistants were being employed to do the bulk of insurance work for inadequate remuneration were still being made in the late 1930s (PEP, 1937, p. 144).

Too Many Patients
Another complaint about contract practice was that doctors were 'compelled' to take more patients than they could efficiently serve. According to the annual report of the chief medical officer at the Ministry of Health for 1919–20, under pre-1911

contract practice the doctor, 'in respect of his working class practice . . . was under constant temptation to undertake the care of patients beyond the number to whom he could give adequate attendance, in order that he might obtain an income suitable for the social position which it was desirable that he should be able to maintain' (MOH, 1919–20, p. 188).

However, under the state scheme the same criticism continued to be voiced. Initially there was no limit on the number of patients that could join a doctor's panel. As a result, some had huge lists. After the 1911 medical benefit scheme had been operating for some years there were still complaints that doctors took too many patients to be able to provide proper attention (see e.g. *Oddfellows Magazine*, August 1918, p. 265). Writing in 1917, Brend thought that many working-class practices were too large. A 'considerable number' of panel doctors without partners or assistants had 2,000 patients, some had 3,000 and some even 4,000. Most also undertook private practice. On the assumption that one insured person had on average one and a half dependants a panel of 2,000 would have meant about 5,000 potential patients.

Brend cites Dr Alfred Salter (in *Medical World*, April 1914) who himself saw 'on average seventy-six cases in the morning and ninety-two in the evening. It worked out at three and a quarter minutes for each patient, one and a quarter of which was taken up in writing.' Patients had to wait on average, two and a half hours, unless they were present at the start. The Cambridge Insurance Committee found that one local doctor, who allowed his dispenser to write prescriptions and give certificates, had made 12,457 consultations and visits in 1914. With private patients the total came to 20,660. Brend claimed he had witnessed over seventy patients being seen by one doctor in three hours. Towards the end of the surgery they were shown in three at a time. A short distance away another doctor had seen less than a dozen patients. This was the result of free choice. People preferred to wait to see the doctor they regarded as best (Brend, 1917, pp. 178–180).

Until 1920 there was no limit to the number of patients a doctor could have on his list. The chief medical officer reported in that year that 'inadequacy of service' had resulted from taking too many patients. As a result a limit of 3,000 was imposed, although local insurance committees could impose lower limits and many did (MOH, 1919–20, p. 195). And in 1924 this figure was reduced to 2,500 for a single doctor, still above that attacked by some doctors as too high in the days before the 1911 scheme.

We have no systematic survey of list sizes in the pre-1911 period. We do have list sizes today. In England in October 1981, the average list size for the 22,304 GPs (unrestricted principals) was 2201. Sizes varied as follows:

TABLE 4 **List Sizes, England, October 1981**

List size	*Number of Practitioners*
Less than 1000	371
1000–1499	1583
1500–1999	5660
2000–2499	8456
2500–2999	4710
3000 plus	1524

SOURCE: DHSS, 1982.

That is, about 7 per cent of doctors had lists of between 3,000 and 3,500 (the maximum size). The original maximum had been 4,000 for sole practitioners, but this had soon been lowered to 3,500 (Eckstein, 1960, p. 68).

Although we cannot compare list sizes before 1913 with list sizes under panel practice and the NHS, we can compare annual average attendance rates. The BMA survey report of 1905 did not provide figures for list sizes in contract practice, but it did provide average attendance figures. The 40,000 subscribers surveyed enjoyed an average of 4.1 attendances from the doctor per year. This is round about the same as post-1948 studies have found (see e.g. Cartwright, 1967, pp. 24–5).

The annual report of the chief medical officer of the Ministry of Health for 1919–20 found that average attendances per annum per head of the total insured population were 'broadly' four during the early years of the scheme (MOH, 1919–20, p. 189). These figures suggest that the crude workload per contract patient was not markedly different on average for any of the three periods: pre-1913, 1913-48, post-1948.

Surgery standards were criticized before 1911, and indeed

before 1946. But these complaints are still being voiced today. In the early days of the NHS there were frequent complaints about the physical condition of surgeries (Brown, 1978, p. 34). Yet the medical institutes, many of which had fine premises, had been displaced in 1948.

The fact that surgery premises continued to be rather poor had often been put down to the fact that doctors had no financial incentive to improve them (see e.g. Brown, 1978, p. 34). This was one of the main reasons for changing the method by which GPs were paid in 1966. Most of their expenditure on rent could be reimbursed, and sharing premises became financially more attractive. However, the Royal Commission on the National Health Service found on their visits that the conditions obtaining in some surgeries 'were clearly unacceptable' (RCNHS, 1979, para. 7.35).

Conclusions

According to Titmuss, the medical profession at the turn of the century was engaged in a 'Hobbesian struggle for independence from the power and authority exercised over their lives, their work and their professional values by voluntary associations and private enterprise.' The battle of the clubs, he thought, was 'fundamentally, a struggle for professional and private freedom' (1959, p. 308).

This struggle, as we have seen, was won by the medical profession with the aid of the ostensibly benevolent state. Moreover, the chief instrument of this victory of producer over consumer – the 1911 Act – was class legislation, deliberately singling out the 'ignorant' manual workers for paternalist compulsion. The doctors argued that consumer dominance meant cheap and nasty medicine – a charge still repeated by today's paternalists – but this claim was false.

It was not true of all contract practice, and above all it was not true of the medical institutes, though some contract practice at any given moment did give consumers grounds for complaint. Yet the principles on which the 1911 scheme was based were those of contract practice: an annual premium in return for medical advice and medicines, supplied free at the time of use. And the medical institutes, which were free from the criticisms habitually directed against contract practice, were deliberately discriminated against. If improved standards had been of paramount importance the medical institutes would have been given an unimpeded role. They were not permitted to play an equal part in the 1911 scheme because the doctors' chief goal was increased power at the expense of consumers. Criticism of standards was one of the weapons used to erect a respectable cover for their real aim: the eradication of competition. Fearing that the doctors would refuse to cooperate with the scheme on their own terms, the government gave them the power they sought.

But above all, criticism of standards did not end with the 1911 Act. The volume of complaint continued loud and clear. These complaints were probably no more justified after 1911 than they were beforehand. There were differences between fee-paying private practice on the one hand and contract practice/panel practice on the other. The chief difference continued to be that a fee bought convenience. It did not, as a rule, purchase more thorough diagnosis and treatment. The behaviour of doctors as a group displays the full gamut of human frailties, but the great majority were honourable men who offered rich and poor alike the same standard of clinical care. The 1911 Act made little or no difference to the real or imagined differences between private fee-paying and pre-paid capitation practice, whether voluntary contract practice or state panel practice.

9
No 'System': The Uninsured

The period from 1913 to 1948 is of particular interest because it makes possible a comparison between market provision and state provision. The working population was covered by the National Insurance scheme, but wives and children were not. They obtained health care in the marketplace. Chapters 9, 10 and 11 describe what arrangements emerged to deliver primary health-care to women and children, and ask whether or not the conclusions drawn for the pre-1911 period can also be drawn for 1913–1948.

The main types of provision were: the outpatient departments of the voluntary hospitals, the free dispensaries, the provident dispensaries, friendly society lodge practice, insurance against medical fees (including friendly society approved panels), public medical services, private doctors' clubs, works clubs, and friendly society medical institutes. The latter, in addition to providing a service for the non-insured population, were also 'approved institutions' under the National Health Insurance scheme and are the subject of a separate chapter.

Hospital Outpatient Departments
Many people continued to use outpatient departments instead of a GP, even though by the 1930s many voluntary hospitals were encouraging or even requiring patients to go to their GP first. In 1935 there were 1,013 voluntary hospitals. They admitted 1.2 million inpatients and attended 5.6 million outpatients (PEP, 1937, p. 231). Some public hospitals also performed a similar role.

The Free and Provident Dispensaries
Free dispensaries financed by charities continued to function in

many large towns. In the mid 1930s there were over twenty in the London area alone.

Provident dispensaries also continued to function. In the London area there were nearly twenty. Among these the Battersea Provident Dispensary was one of the largest with over 6,000 members in 1936. Single persons paid 3d a week. The panel of doctors received a capitation fee of 6s (PEP, 1937, p. 152).

Private Doctors' Clubs
A number of these clubs continued to function, but it is impossible to estimate how many persons were covered. In the judgement of the BMA survey of 1938–9 it was evident that private clubs were 'gradually dying out'. In the 'great majority' of cases divisional secretaries reported that there were no private clubs. Often they had been absorbed into public medical services. Rates tended to be at least 3d a week, although local practices varied enormously (BMA, General Practice Committee, Documents 1938–9, GP107, pp. 1–6). It seems unlikely that more than 100,000 persons were covered by private club membership.

Works or Shop Clubs
Many factories and all collieries provided medical attendance. Some were managed by the employer and some by committees representing employees. In Scotland many had broken down due to unemployment, but unemployment clubs had emerged to continue medical attendance for those out of work (PEP, 1937, p. 150). Usually such schemes covered families as well as employees. PEP felt unable to estimate the numbers covered, but we know that there were still about one million miners in the mid 1930s. Their dependants must have accounted for at least another two to two and a half million people.

Public Medical Services
The BMA had been promoting the establishment of 'public medical services'. The largest was in London, and by 1937 throughout the country there were 'just below eighty' services with 650,000 subscribers. A survey of fifty-one of these found that for each subscription 1.86 persons were 'at risk'. On this basis a total of about 1.2 million people were covered by public medical services. About 4,000 doctors were involved. Capita-

tion fees averaged 11s 2d, with large towns more expensive than rural areas (*BMJ* Supplement, 10 December 1938, pp. 357–62). Expansion in the 1930s had been rapid. In 1932 there had been only thirty-two public medical services.

In the 1930s the London Public Medical Service set up the London Public Medical Service Extension to provide for non-insured middle class patients at higher capitation rates. Three different rates applied in London: £4 per family of four for incomes between £250 and £375; £4 10s for incomes between £375 and £475; and £5 for incomes from £475 to £550 (PEP, 1937, pp. 153–4). Included in the service was an annual 'overhaul' for preventive purposes (BMA, Medico-Political Committee, Documents 1936–7, MP75).

The Essex Public Medical service had 34,156 members in 1938. There were 305 participating doctors (*BMJ* Supplement, 12 August 1939). Some of the public medical services were being run in conjunction with the friendly societies and some were not. The Oxford public medical service was one organized with friendly society cooperation. Adults paid 12s a year and juveniles 9s 6d. When the friendly societies collected the contribution 5 per cent was deducted for administration. To resolve problems between the doctors and the friendly societies a joint standing committee had been established (*BMJ* Supplement, 1937, vol. 1, p. 241). These rates were lower than those desired by the BMA, which was particularly insistent that juvenile rates should not be lower than adult fees. The friendly societies, in return for these lower rates, agreed not to enter into contracts with doctors for different fees.

Perhaps the most successful of the public medical services was the Leicester public medical service. This had originated as the Leicester and Leicestershire Provident Dispensary in 1833. By 1911 the organization had 90,000 members served by ten branch dispensaries. When the National Insurance Act was passed the managers decided to close down, but a group of Leicester doctors felt there was still a need to provide for the uninsured wives and children. In 1912 the Leicester public medical service was born. About 50,000 persons continued to use the service, and the number of branch dispensaries expanded to thirteen. Specialist services – opthalmic, aural, radiological, and dental – were approved at reduced fees. By the late 1930s doctors were paid 6s per annum for attendance only. Disabled and blind members paid no contribution, but doctors were paid 6s a year by the public medical service for each such person on their list. Relations with the friendly societies were very close, including Leicester's two medical institutes. Doctors were paid for insured and uninsured friendly society members through the public medical service. The Foresters Medical Association and Dispensary, for instance, functioned through the public medical service thereby offering its members a free choice from among the seventy doctors on the panel. Closely associated with the public medical service was a 25-bed hospital, opened in 1903 on the initiative of the provident dispensary, and a maternity hospital, opened two years later, also by the board of the provident dispensary. When it closed in 1948 the public medical service had around 60,000 members (private papers of F.A. Alexander, Leicester Medical Society Library).

Friendly Society Lodge Practice
According to Titmuss, 'With the withdrawal of the working-classes, club and contract practice virtually collapsed after 1911' (1959, p. 307). This was an exaggeration. Most of those who had been covered by lodge practice before 1911 were covered by National Insurance, and so the number of persons obtaining medical aid did decline drastically. But the lodges continued to provide for those members not covered by National Insurance. They included not only women and children but also a considerable number of male friendly society members who 'accidentally' got left out of National Insurance. According to Lloyd George, the original plan had been to extend friendly society membership to every working person. It was not anticipated that some existing friendly society members would be worse off. But they were. It became necessary to pass an Amending Act in 1913 to include two groups of persons: (a) aged or permanently disabled friendly society members not insured under the Act; and (b) those joining National Insurance who were aged fifty to sixty-five. They were entitled to reduced benefits of 5s to 6s sick pay without medical benefit or 4s to 4s 6d with medical benefit. Under the 1913 National Insurance Amendment Act they were to be allowed 10s sick pay with medical benefit (National Insur-

ance Act (1911) Amendment Bill, *Memorandum on the General Objects of the Bill*, Cd 6914, July 1913).

Friendly societies still trying to provide medical care for members not covered by National Insurance, found that the National Insurance Act turned the old much-admired friendly society doctor into a different individual. It brought the emergence of the 'commercial medical man'. For the elderly and other friendly society members excluded from the state insurance scheme doctors demanded increases from around 4s to 9s. Unless their societies or branches were able to help, some members were forced to turn to the Poor Law (*Foresters Miscellany*, May 1914, pp. 132–3). Not all doctors behaved selfishly. Some continued to serve elderly friendly society members at the old rates (*Foresters Miscellany*, May 1914, p. 133).

However, by the mid 1930s relations between the friendly societies and the BMA had improved as the friendly societies adjusted themselves to the realities of the doctors' state-imposed monopoly power. In some areas doctors and lodges cooperated to establish medical services for non-insured persons. The Independent Order of Rechabites had made arrangements for its juvenile members in about a hundred towns involving 350 doctors. In Leeds, 150 doctors served 14,000 juvenile members of the Independent Order of Oddfellows, Kingston Unity friendly society. The children paid 2d per week, or 6s 6d per year (PEP, 1937, p. 150). And an agreement came into effect in 1921 for uninsured members in Montgomery. Adults paid 15s per annum and juniors 10s, for both attendance and drugs (*Oddfellows Magazine*, February 1921, p. 40).

According to the BMA's surveys of contract practice rates carried out in 1935–6 and 1938–9, contract practice to adult members of friendly societies was 'steadily diminishing'. But it was still to be found in many areas. Rates varied a good deal, depending on competition. In 1935–6, the annual fee in Bath was 5s; in Birmingham, 11s; in Chesterfield, 13s; Norwich, 12s; Kent, 6s; and in Barnsley, 10s. The highest was 16s, in Ely (BMA, Medico-Political Committee, Documents, 1936–7, MP31, pp. 14–18).

The BMA surveys of 1935–6 and 1938–9 were incomplete, but the BMA believed that 90 per cent of existing contract schemes had been covered. The surveys were concerned with rates of pay and not the numbers insured, but some indications are provided. Combined with the figures published by the Registrar of Friendly Societies, we can estimate the number of people obtaining medical care through the friendly societies.

In 1930 there were 700 purely juvenile friendly societies with 185,000 members. Friendly societies with branches had 2,982,000 members; dividing societies, 499,000; and friendly societies without branches paying sick benefit on accumulating principles had 1,152,000 members. Not all these members were insured for medical care, and many were covered by National Insurance but had opted to take out additional voluntary sickness or other insurance. The deposit societies offered co-insurance and I have therefore considered them separately below. The 185,000 members of the juvenile societies would have been covered for medical care, and in the 1930s the number insured was increasing rapidly. In 1935 membership was 214,000. The friendly societies with branches had 134,000 members aged under sixteen in 1930; the sickness benefit societies (on accumulating principles) had 122,000; and the dividing societies, 5,000; a total of 446,000 juvenile members. The societies with branches had 2,189,000 members aged over sixteen; the accumulating societies, 947,000; and the dividing societies 370,000. Of the total adult membership of 3,506,000 the majority of women members would have subscribed for medical care. The Registrar did not publish separate figures for male and female members, but the evidence of the NCFS to the Beveridge committee of 1942 suggests that females comprised between a quarter and fifth of total voluntary membership. (In 1941, 1.1 million out of 4.6 million were females, i.e. 24 per cent.) (PRO PIN8/88.) On this formula, of the 3.5 million adult voluntary members in 1935 around 700,000 were women. If only three quarters of these obtained medical care through the lodges, this suggests a figure of over 520,000. Some of the male members would also have attended lodge doctors. If only 10 per cent did so this suggests a figure of about 280,000. All told, at least somewhere in the region of 1.2 million persons must have been obtaining medical care through friendly societies other than deposit societies in the mid 1930s.

Insurance Against Medical Fees

After the 1911 Act some friendly societies developed new schemes for insurance against the payment of doctors' fees. Some medical schemes provided for repayment of the whole fee, and some for part. In some cases any doctor could be consulted and a repayment of whatever fee he charged claimed. In most cases a doctor had to be selected from a panel of doctors who had agreed to charge specified fees.

On the introduction of National Insurance in 1911 the South London District of the Manchester Unity established a fee-for-service scheme. Members initially contributed 1d a week (soon increased to 2d) into a common fund, the district medical aid fund. Members could consult any doctor, pay the bill and recover the sum from the fund. Doctors charged 3s 0d per home visit and 2s 0d for a surgery consultation. By 1925 there were 6,000 subscribers to the financially successful scheme. Over the twelve years average annual expenditure had been about £2,000 (*Oddfellows Magazine*, May 1925, pp. 256–7). Such 'medical pools' as they were often called, were also successful in some other areas, such as Swadlincote, Coalville, and Wolverton, but their success had only been accomplished by placing a limit on the amounts doctors were permitted to charge (*Foresters Miscellany*, May 1923, pp. 214–5).

Not all of the similar fee-for-service funds succeeded. When the 1911 Act came into force, thirty of the 800 existing members of the Old Elm Tree Lodge in Chipping Norton, who had been entitled to medical care under the previous arrangement, were excluded. The lodge had established a medical aid fund for them, but in 1925 it was losing money (*Oddfellows Magazine*, April 1925, p. 206). In London the AOF began a pooling scheme for their members. Each contributor paid 5s per year, and the London United District of the AOF paid an additional £1,000 into the fund. Doctors charged 1s 6d per surgery consultation and 2s 6d per home visit. However, within fifteen months the whole fund was facing a debt of £500. This was attributed to the considerable 'over-servicing' practised by doctors. The scheme had to be wound up (*Foresters Miscellany*, March 1913, p. 108; *Foresters Miscellany*, May 1914, p. 133).

Those schemes run on part-payment principles (co-insurance), however, expanded very rapidly. In 1936, over 1.3 million members of the National Deposit Friendly Society (NDFS) were covered for payment of a proportion of doctors' bills, as were 57,000 members of the Teachers Provident Society (PEP, 1937, p. 154).

Until 1948, under the NDFS system members paid 2s 6d for a surgery attendance and 3s 6d for a home visit, including medicine. Payment could be made direct to the doctor or to the member (NDFS, *Rules*, 1949, rule 91). For male members who had joined between the ages of sixteen and thirty, 75 per cent of the doctor's fee was paid by the society. Fc: those who joined between ages five to sixteen or thirty to forty, the society paid two thirds. The remainder was paid from the member's personal deposit account which the society held in return for interest paid to the member (ibid., rule 87). However, according to the BMA, a 'considerable number' of doctors accepted the NDFS payment alone in full settlement of the account (BMA, Medico-Political Committee, Documents 1936–7, MP75).

It was not only the friendly societies that offered insurance against fees. The BMA surveyed a number of organizations in the field in 1936. There was the Anchor Doctors' Bills Policy at Lloyds, operated through Family Medical Services Ltd; the Sickness Insurance Company Ltd, which charged 15s a month for the whole family and included both GP and hospital care; the Scottish Clerks Association; the Manchester Warehousemen and Clerks Provident Association; the Mutual Health Insurance Society of Richmond; and the Secondary, Technical, and University Teachers Insurance Society (BMA, Medico-Political Committee, Documents, 1936–7, MP75).

10
'Approved Institutions': Medical Institutes after the 1911 Act

At one stage the government planned to permit the medical institutes no place at all in the medical benefit scheme. But during the debate on the Bill the friendly societies sought to persuade the government to allow them a role. The Friendly Societies Medical Alliance reasoned that the government was going to make use of doctors and chemists, who offered their services for 'profit and gain'. Why not, they asked, also permit non-profit friendly societies to offer medical care? It was true that some doctors were outspoken against the friendly societies, but those who were most loud in their condemnation of medical institutes were not currently serving as lodge doctors. Some of these critics would have been unacceptable to the friendly societies, and others would have left contract practice for private practice and had no wish to return. Why, asked the friendly society leaders, when the medical institutes were employing many doctors on perfectly amicable terms, should they have to satisfy other doctors who had no connection with the friendly societies? (*Oddfellows Magazine*, August 1911, p. 520; July 1911, p. 355)

It looked as if the medical institutes were to be excluded when luck came to their aid. In July 1911 a by-election was held in the Luton constituency, home of the Luton Friendly Societies Medical Institute, one of the most successful of the institutes. The by-election campaign enabled the friendly societies to press their case, and pledges to support the medical institutes were obtained from both candidates. The victor was Cecil Harmsworth who, true to his word, moved a successful amendment to the National Insurance Bill which gave the medical institutes a role in the administration of medical benefit. They were allowed to register as 'approved institutions' under the Act. Also entitled to register were the Welsh medical aid societies, the works clubs run largely by miners. Had it not been for the fortuitous by-election it may well have been the end for the medical institutes (Pride, 1923).

But the Harmsworth amendment was a small concession, and the Bill as amended in August 1911 represented a serious defeat for the friendly societies. The main disadvantage of the Bill, in the judgement of friendly society leaders, was that it required acceptance of *one* scheme. There was insufficient room for local variation. And the *one* scheme was that preferred by the BMA. At a special meeting of the FSMA in September 1911, delegates said they felt as if the BMA had captured the government (*Oddfellows Magazine*, October 1911, p. 584). But the friendly societies were slow to react. They had, in the judgement of the grand master of Manchester Unity, been resting on the justice of their case while the BMA had been lobbying vigorously. The friendly societies, he urged, should redouble their efforts, for as a result of BMA propaganda MPs were appallingly ignorant of the truth (*Oddfellows Magazine*, November 1911, p. 629). But by then it was already too late.

Fortunately the Harmsworth amendment to the Bill did permit some kind of role for the medical institutes as well as for the Welsh medical aid societies. But on the insistence of the BMA, medical institutes were allowed into the scheme on terms highly unfavourable to their development. Under section 15(4) of the 1911 Act, friendly society medical institutes in existence in December 1911 were allowed to offer medical benefits to persons insured under the Act, subject to the approval of the local insurance committee and the Insurance Commission. This not only put a maximum limit on the number of medical institutes, as the BMA had intended; it also put the institutes at the mercy of local insurance committees, with their strong professional representation. Doctors, by comparison, had an entitlement to join the scheme if they wished. At an advisory committee meeting in June 1912 the FSMA urged that this approval should not rest 'on the caprice of any local committee'. The 'ground of efficiency or non-efficiency', they said, 'should be the only ground'.

And if qualified doctors were employed by the institutes, they like any others should be entitled to participate. Robert Morant, who chaired this meeting, curtailed the discussion of the future of the medical institutes. He was plainly hostile (PRO PIN2/19, pp. 36-41).

The commissioners, and later the Ministry of Health, continued to prevent the formation of new medical institutes or to allow existing ones to extend. The National Conference of Friendly Societies pressed regularly for this disability to be removed, but to no avail. However, sect on 15(3) allowed insured persons to make their 'own collective arrangements' and a very few new schemes had been established in South Wales under this section. The Royal Commission called this an evasion of section 15(4) and urged that the loophole be closed (as indeed it was, by the 1928 National Health Insurance Act) (RCNHI, 1926, *Report*, p. 263).

In 1924 the rules governing the procedures for changing doctors were liberalized. But medical institutes were deliberately excluded from the liberalization. From 1924 the insured person could transfer from one panel practitioner to another by simple presentation of their medical card to the doctor of their choice. But to transfer either from or to a medical institute, it was necessary for the insured person to give notice before 1 June or 1 December for transfer on the 1 July or 1 January following. The friendly societies argued for equal treatment for persons wanting to transfer to or from medical institutes, a request supported by the Federation Committee of the English, Scottish and Welsh Associations of Insurance Committees (*Medical Benefit Regulations*, 1924, regulation 16(1) and (2); RCNHI, 1926, *Appendices*, Appendix XXXVI). But they got nowhere. Not only was the number of medical institutes limited to those in existence at the time of the Act, they were also subject to discrimination from the very beginning. Most notably, they were not paid on the same basis as panel practitioners, with the result that approved institutions were paid less per capita than panel doctors. One of the arguments used for treating the institutes differently was that they also treated non-insured persons, and so the Ministry had to ensure that money from the Insurance Fund was not used to support services to the uninsured. But the same applied to panel practitioners. Many also carried out private practice, and many also had private clubs which catered for the dependants of insured persons. They, however, were subject to no additional regulation.

Payments to approved institutions were made from a special fund, the Institutions Fund, not per capita but according to the principle that insurance committees could pay up to a maximum sum subject to being satisfied that payments did not exceed the amounts actually expended by the medical institutes on medical care of insured members. This was initially interpreted by the Insurance Commissioners to require an investigation into the non-insured as well as the insured side of each institute. Under Circular 163/IC an apportionment of costs was to be made, and institutes to be paid this sum. Doctors were paid a per capita allowance, but medical institutes found themselves subject to an investigation before they were paid, with the result that they were often paid less. This made it more difficult for the institutes to lay aside funds for epidemics, or for the improvement of their premises, or for the extension of their range of services. It was, therefore, more difficult for them to keep up their earlier rate of improvement.

Obstacles were also put in the way of patients opting for medical care through the friendly societies. When the scheme began, ordinarily a pink ticket was signed by the insured person, but patients opting to join a medical institute were made to fill in an additional form. To make matters worse an official error was made with the original form and so members were required to fill in a further document (*Oddfellows Magazine*, July 1913, p. 538). The FSMA pressed in vain for equal treatment: 'We do not ask, or desire, preferential treatment,' said the FSMA, 'but in the name of common sense and justice, we should have equality' (*Foresters Miscellany*, June 1913, pp. 210–11).

After protests by the FSMA it was agreed that from August 1913 the capitation rate would be paid on production of a certificate declaring that the amount spent had been equivalent to the capitation rate multiplied by the number of insured members. This agreement lasted until the end of 1919 (RCNHI, 1926, Appendices, p. 90). But from January 1920 the capitation fee was increased from 9s to 11s. This increase was not paid to medical institutes. They were required, unlike ordinary panel doctors, to show that they had spent this amount. After further protests, it was agreed to divide their expenditure on insured and non-insured persons and to pay them the amount expended on their insured members. But the division did not depend on their actual expenditure, instead it was paid according to a formula. In the Glamorgan Insurance Committee area the formula was that three sevenths of the total expenditure on medical benefit for all members was deemed to have been expended on insured members (RCNHI, 1926, Appendices, pp. 92, 4154). In the event the Glamorgan Insurance Committee found on examination of society accounts that they spent 'considerably in excess' per insured person than the capitation fee (RCNHI, 1926, Q. 13320).

The ordinary panel doctor did not necessarily receive the exact capitation fee. It was adjusted to take account of emergency treatment provided for other panel doctors. But it was not adjusted, as it was for medical institutes, to take into account expenditure on treating the non-insured. Unlike the panel doctors, medical institutes also received no share of the unallocated insured person's fund. Each year an allocation was made for all insured persons who had not put their name on a list. A sum was paid to panel doctors to cover treatment of insured persons not on their list. The medical institutes received no such payment, though they did treat unallocated persons (RCNHI, 1926, Qs 16394–16400).

In addition, the institutes were treated differently over the war allowance paid to other panel doctors for the additional costs they incurred during the war years. Doctors whose net income from all sources did not exceed £500 per annum were paid an extra 12½ per cent of the insurance fees normally payable. Medical institutes were not treated systematically in the same manner, although payments were made to some (*Foresters Miscellany*, May 1919, p. 194: *Oddfellows Magazine*, July 1921, p. 481: PRO MH81/64).

Throughout the life of the scheme the BMA kept the Ministry of Health under constant pressure to discriminate against approved institutions. In March 1921, for instance, Alfred Cox, on behalf of the BMA, wrote to the ministry complaining that the Norwich FSMI was charging 3s per quarter for juvenile members. They felt this was too low and accused the institute of subsidizing juveniles out of their income from the National

Insurance scheme. Not satisfied with the ministry's initial reply, Cox wrote again on 22 April emphasizing that the BMA 'strongly objects' to the subsidization of the non-insured. R.W. Harris replied, saying that he could not carry on the correspondence on an official footing but proposed a private chat when Cox was next in the ministry. On 7 May Cox met Harris, who made a note of the BMA's reasoning: 'From the BMA point of view it is particularly important that the assumption that these uninsured juveniles can be treated for the same charge as an insured person should not be established as a precedent which might be used in the event of the extension of GP treatment to the general population' (PRO MH81/54). Even at this early date the BMA was taking all necessary measures to maximize the cash take doctors could extract from the government in the event of an extension of medical benefit.

The Friendly Societies Medical Alliance put its case for equal treatment to the Royal Commission. Complaints about discrimination were not only made by the Friendly Societies Medical Alliance (RCNHI, 1926, Appendix LIII) but also by the Friendly Societies Medical Officers Union, which represented fifty of the sixty medical officers working in FSMA affiliated medical institutes. The organization's evidence was partly critical of medical institutes and partly supportive, and under questioning differences of view emerged between the three representatives of the association who appeared before the Royal Commission. But they referred to 'repressive regulations' which had starved some institutes to death. They particularly complained about the Coventry Provident Dispensary, by that time a friendly society affiliate, which, they said, was 'still struggling against misrepresentations and injustices which clog their activities and threaten their existence' (ibid., Appendix LIV, para. 5). The union complained that regulations were either interpreted in a hostile manner when convenient or, if the regulations were not open to hostile interpretation, they were not applied at all (ibid., para. 8(3)). As a result of this discrimination by the Ministry, medical officers felt they had to 'submit to underpayment'.

Complaints were also made by the South Wales and Monmouthshire Alliance of Medical Aid Societies. They supported the FSMA viewpoint and complained that in their area insurance committees had even attempted to interfere with funds obtained from non-government sources. They strongly complained about their non-representation on the insurance committees, on the medical committees (which laid down the conditions under which doctors would practise) and on the medical service sub-committees, which handled complaints against doctors.

The BMA claimed that medical institutes offered inferior service. Though no evidence was adduced in support of this view, the Royal Commission repeated these claims. However, they did rather grudgingly conclude that there was no justification for recommending the closure of the institutes on account of the standard of service offered (RCNHI, 1926, *Report*, pp. 261–2). They had in fact been presented with considerable evidence that the medical institutes had provided a standard of service which was much higher than that being offered by the government (see e.g. Appendix LV, appendix; Appendix LIII, appendix; Qs 16415, 16423, 16559–60).

In 1926 there were two medical institutes at Leicester, one in 'very fine' premises and both offering consulting rooms superior to those of the average GP. There were close ties with the Leicester public medical service, with which all the doctors in Leicester were involved (RCNHI, 1926, Qs 6369–72). In 1927 the largest of the institutes was the Norwich Friendly Societies Medical Institute, which provided for about one seventh of the population of that city (*Foresters Miscellany*, June 1927, p. 291). The Glamorgan Insurance Committee testified that a range of additional benefits were being supplied free by medical aid societies in their area: dental treatment, maternity services, nursing, an ambulance car, rail fares for hospital patients, contributions paid to hospitals and convalescent homes, major and minor operations, artificial limbs and appliances in addition to those supplied under the insurance scheme (RCNHI, 1926, Appendix XXXIX, para. 13).

The Tredegar Workmen's Medical Aid Society and five of the other societies in Wales provided a cottage hospital in which the medical officers could carry out all necessary operations. The South Wales and Monmouthshire Alliance of Medical Aid Societies represented sixteen institutes. There were three others in their area not affiliated. The institutes were funded chiefly by

paypacket deductions paid by the men in the mines and steelworks. Other workmen and individuals also contributed. In
total the Alliance provided for 105,000 persons and offered a
standard of service well in excess of that being provided by the
National Insurance scheme (ibid., see Appendix LV).

In its evidence to the Royal Commission, the BMA expressed
hostility to medical institutes, and especially to the arrangements prevailing in South Wales which were based on mines and
steelworks. In particular they objected that the institutes were
not guided in medical matters by a purely medical committee, as
the insurance committees were guided by the panel committees
(RCNHI, 1926, Appendix XLVII, para. 44 and appendix B). It
is clear from their evidence that the BMA's objection to medical
institutes was lay control, and nothing else (RCNHI, 1926, Q.
15290). In giving evidence that the institutes in the mining areas of
South Wales had been 'very detrimental indeed' to the medical
service given in those areas Dr Cox, Medical Secretary of the
BMA, said, in typically caustic style, that they proceeded on 'entirely wrong lines, the theory being that the miner, who is of
course a very politically-minded person and who believes that he
is able to manage services of all kinds, thought that he could
manage the doctor' (RCNHI, 1926, Q. 15222).

One of the results of the BMA's barrage of complaint about
lay control, was that members of the Royal Commission seem to
have looked upon lay control as an automatically bad thing. But
leaving aside the desirability or otherwise of lay control, there
was no lay control of clinical judgements in the medical institutes. Doctors were not told what to do by institute organizers,
although in the event of a member's complaint, they might have
to explain their conduct. In panel practice there was also lay control in the form of the government and the local committees.
And in practice the government did interfere with clinical judgements. A number of doctors were surcharged for 'extravagant
prescribing', something that did not happen in the institutes. In
the institutes doctors were given the 'fullest liberty' (RCNHI,
1926, Q. 16878).

Moreover, when complaints were made against doctors, the
Minister was the final judge. So it could not be said that the issue
at stake was straightforwardly for or against lay control. The
issue was what form should the complaints machinery take? The

BMA wanted it to be remote and ineffective; not close at hand and effective. The complaints machinery of the institutes was often more effective than that of the insurance committees. This was because the final say lay with neither the doctors nor patients, but with impartial arbitrators in whose selection patients had a say. The BMA's view was the same some years later when hospital reform was under discussion. The BMA opposed local authority control, but favoured control through a centralized ministry which they could capture or manipulate.

Medical Institutes and the Uninsured

One of the criticisms of pre-1911 club practice was that women and children were often not included. Ironically, government National Insurance did not include them either. But not only did the 1911 medical benefit scheme exclude women; it put obstacles in the way of extending non-government provision for them. Up to 1911 the friendly societies were steadily expanding provision for women and children through the medical institutes. The 1911 Act seriously inhibited their continued development.

Nevertheless the medical institutes did continue to provide a service for the non-insured as well as those insured under the 1911 Act. In 1915 the Luton FSMI was being run jointly by the AOF and Manchester Unity branches along with the Luton Industry Friendly Society. Confinements cost 15s; minor surgery – such as the removal of tonsils and adenoids – cost 10s; no extra charge was made for treatment of fractures, dislocations, cuts, burns, bruises and blood poisoning. Vaccinations cost 1s 6d, but diptheria and 'other serums and anti-toxins' were provided free. Other surgery was available at a fee to be approved by the committee.

By 1915, when male members of the York FSMI were covered by National Insurance, the subscription was 6s for wives and 3s for children under 16. Widows and orphans could continue their membership. Other dependent relatives were provided for at the same rate as wives. For confinements a fee of 15s was payable. One of the largest institutes at that time was the Coventry Dispensary. In 1916 it had 7,158 members (RFS, *Annual Report*, 1918). In the early years the medical institutes had paid fixed salaries, but during the twentieth century many paid their doctors according to the number of patients under their care (FSMA, *Annual Report*, 1944, in PRO MH77/94).

By 1924, forty-four medical institutes were affiliated to the FSMA. They had 120,000 insured members, with an additional 41,000 uninsured adults receiving attendance, plus 60,000 juveniles (RCNHI, 1926, Q. 16,349). In 1929 the FSMA had 142,000 voluntary members in addition to its 106,000 state members. By 1937 state membership was 119,000. On the eve of the NHS it was 100,000 (NCFS, *Annual Reports*, 1930, 1938, 1948).

The Cost of Discrimination
The number of institutes declined steadily after the 1911 Act but membership increased. New institutes were forbidden to become approved institutions under the Act and, although it was permissible for new institutes to be established for the uninsured population, it was very difficult to run a financially viable service without providing a service for the breadwinner as well as dependants. There was pressure to establish new institutes. Indeed, new medical schemes were being planned right up to the eve of the NHS. In December 1945, for example, a group of individuals in Slough were planning to establish a new medical institute. They wrote to the ministry asking if their scheme would clash with the government's own plans. The reply, in January 1946, suggested that they defer their scheme until the government announced their plan (PRO MH77/93). This institute was never established, but after 1913 several new medical institutes were founded. They could not, however, become approved institutions and so their development was stifled.

The discrimination against them cost the existing medical institutes dear. In England in 1910 there were about a hundred medical institutes with around 350,000 members. Under half of these members were not covered by the National Insurance Act and continued to be shown in the returns of the Registrar of Friendly Societies after 1913. The official figures showed only voluntary members. Those compulsorily insured under the Act do not appear in the Registrar's figures from 1913 onwards. This explains the drop from 311,878 members in 1912, to 138,578 in 1913. Most of the difference (173,300 members) represents persons who could have been covered by the Act. Unfortunately we do not have a figure for the number of members of approved institutions until 1924. We do know that in England alone, between 1911 and 1924, thirty-four approved institutions closed, usually by transferring their premises to their existing medical officers. By 1924 there were only fifty-two approved institutions with a total of 135,000 insured members approved under section 15(4) [24(4)]. Forty-four of these, with 120,000 members, were affiliated to the FSMA (RCNHI, 1926, Q. 16,349). Many closed during the first year of the scheme because of the obstacles put in their way by the insurance committees. The most serious problem was that no income was received from the government until after October 1913. By this time no income had been received from insured persons since June 1912, and the scheme had been in operation since January 1913 (RCNHI, 1926, Qs 16,356–9).

From these figures we can estimate the loss of medical institute members due to official discrimination. In 1910 there were eighty-five registered societies with 329,450 members. We have no figure for 1911, but in 1912 there were eighty-eight registered societies with 311,878 members. Thus by the end of 1912, by which time registration for the medical benefit scheme had been under way since June, some losses were already being experienced, although the number of registered institutes increased. There had long been a number of unregistered institutes, and it may be that they registered in 1911 or 1912 in order to increase their chances of being approved under section 15(4). If the voluntary membership in 1913 is subtracted from the figure for 1910 this provides a rough indication of the potential number of insured persons: 190,000. In 1924 there were about 135,000 insured members, and so we may estimate the membership loss to be around 50,000.

There were no approved institutions in Scotland, but in Wales in the first year of the medical benefit scheme there were forty-two approved institutions covering 56,742 members. By 1914 there were only twenty approved institutions catering for 27,971 members (ICW, 1912–13, p. 658; ICW, 1913–14, p. 572). In 1917 there were fifteen approved institutions with 28,310 members (NHIJC, 1917, p. 338).

In Wales in 1924 there were three medical institutes registered under section 24(3) of the 1924 Act (formerly section 15(3) of the 1911 Act) with a total of 7,431 members; and twelve registered under section 24(4) with 31,225 members (RCNHI, 1926,

Appendices, p. 171). By 1938 there were still twelve approved institutions under what had become section 38(2) of the National Health Insurance Act of 1936 (MOH, Annual Report, 1938–9).

In 1936 118,902 insured persons in England and 33,704 in Wales were receiving medical benefit from medical institutes. In 1945 there were thirty-seven approved institutes in England serving 105,000 members (PRO MH77/93). In 1944 in Wales there were eleven approved institutions with 37,000 members (FSMA, *Annual Report*, 1945, in PRO MH77/94).

In 1947 in England there were forty-nine registered societies with 165,000 members, but this increase is largely explained by the decision of the Great Western Railway Medical Fund Society with 40,000 members to register as a friendly society and join the FSMA. The underlying membership trend during the war was down. These figures are for the medical institutes registered under the Friendly Societies Acts. In addition there were a few unregistered societies, with perhaps another 10,000 members (RFS, *Annual Reports*).

Embryo Health Centres?

By the time of the Royal Commission of 1926, health centres formed an important part of the BMA's plans for health care. Indeed all progressive opinion was in favour of health centres, with the greater possibilities they were believed to offer for consultation between GPs, and for the provision of improved diagnostic aids and specialist care. Ironically, the medical institutes, so mistrusted by the BMA and the Ministry of Health, were health centres in embryo, as at least one member of the Royal Commission had noted. But this made little difference to the generally hostile attitude adopted by the Royal Commission (RCNHI, 1926, Qs 6369–81). It had shown little sympathy for medical institutes from the outset, as the questioning of the Independent Order of Rechabites fairly early in their proceedings indicates (RCNHI, 1926, Qs 6316–59).

The PEP report of 1937 had also noticed that medical institutes were embryo health centres. It described two of the medical institutes it happened to stumble across as providing a comprehensive medical service 'which should be the model of any national system of medical services'. The two services were the Great Western Railway Medical Fund society of Swindon, and the Llanelly and District Medical Service. The latter service had

TABLE 5 **Medical Institutes in England 1870–1947**

Year	Medical Institutes	Membership
1870	2	?
1874	4	?
1883*	32	139,482
1885*	42	211,041
1909*	31	283,983
1910**	85	329,450
National Insurance		
1912**	88	311,878
1913**	79	138,578
1914**	72	144,275
1916**	74	130,652
1920**	64	135,274
1926**	63	148,021
1928**	63	143,181
1929**	66	147,300
1932**	68	145,620
1936**	62	145,188
1937**	60	144,514
1947**	49	165,804

Notes: * numbers affiliated to the FSMA.
       ** medical societies registered as friendly societies in the UK (all in fact in England)

SOURCES: RFS, *Annual Report*, 1911, p. 41; 1918; 1930; 1937; 1938; *Statistical Summaries Friendly Societies, Orders and Branches*, various years; RCNHI, 1926, Q. 16349.

TABLE 6 **Approved Institutions in England 1913–1945**

Year	Number	Membership
1913	?	?
1920	57	?
1924	52	135,000
1930	53	?
1940	41	?
1945	37	105,000

SOURCE: PRO MH77/93

18,100 subscribers (PEP, 1937, pp. 151–2). The Great Western Railway Medical Fund Society at Swindon had been established in 1847. In 1944 it had fourteen full-time medical officers and consultants, plus visiting consultants; three full-time dental surgeons; and a 42-bed hospital with a large outpatient department. It catered for 40,205 persons, around half the population of Swindon. Of these 15,386 were covered by National Insurance (PRO MH77/93).

Other medical institutes also continued to thrive until the NHS was founded. The Norwich FSMI had been founded in 1872. In May 1944 it had four full-time medical officers, two qualified chemists, one dispenser and one assistant, in addition to clerical staff and a receptionist. The city was divided into four districts for home visits, each served by a particular doctor. When specialist consultations were required the institute paid 50 per cent of the fee. The institute was managed by a committee, but 'clinical work was left to the clinician' (PRO MH77/93). As late as October 1947 the institute still had 13,746 members, of which 9,161 were covered by National Insurance. Hours of business were also more attractive than those offered by many panel practitioners. In the 1930s the institute was even open on Christmas Day and Good Friday from 9.30–10.00 a.m. for urgent cases (PRO MH81/54; *Eastern Daily Press*, 19 March 1948).

In 1946, 22,800 people out of the total population of 24,000 were members of the Tredegar Workmen's Medical Aid Society. Miners and steelworkers paid 2d in the £1, and other members 18s a year. The society employed five doctors, one surgeon, two pharmacists, one masseuse (physiotherapist), a dentist and assistant, and a district nurse. For 4d a week 'free' hospital treatment was also available. Glasses could be obtained for 2s 6d, and false teeth at less than cost price. Artificial limbs were free, as were injections, patent foods, drugs, wigs and X-rays. For those who had to go to hospital, a car was provided to the railway station and first-class rail fare paid. The doctors were paid according to their list size, and usually earned about £380 a year. Private patients were allowed, but only about 5 per cent of the population remained outside the medical aid society. It was managed by thirty delegates, mostly miners – the dreaded 'committee' of A.J. Cronin's *The Citadel*.

The classical intellectual's view of the 'ignorant' workers'

efforts to organize their own health care scheme has been as suc-
cinctly expressed as anywhere in A.J. Cronin's best-selling
novel, *The Citadel* (1936). Cronin describes the time he spent in
the 1920s as medical officer to the Aberalaw (Tredegar) medical
aid association. He resigned in protest at the trouble he had had
in persuading the committee, or rather a faction within the committee led by the egregious Ed Chenkin, that it was worthwhile
pursuing his research into miners' diseases. Cronin wrote:

> It was a wonderful ideal, this group of working men controlling the
> medical services of the community for the benefit of their fellow work-
> ers. But it was only an ideal. They were too biased, too unintelligent
> ever to administer such a scheme progressively. It was perpetual
> labour for Owen to drag them along the road with him (1936, p. 179).

Yet Dr Manson (Cronin) had won the day with the assistance
of Owen, the association secretary, who was one of those working-class leaders who dedicated his life to the education and
improvement of his fellows. After winning the vote in committee Manson resigned, not because he had in any sense failed to
win the argument, for he had won convincingly, but because he
was too arrogant to bother spending his time persuading people
he looked down on. His ungrateful decision was accepted and,
when he left, the whole town turned out to say goodbye; and the
men sang 'Men of Harlech' as he departed.

Cronin's portrayal of working-class institutions as 'fine in
principle but dreadful in practice because of the ignorance of the
masses' has been influential (it is occasionally cited by
academics, e.g. Klein, 1973, p. 73) and has always had a strong
appeal to Fabian socialists. The great ideal of the Webbs and
others was that the workers should have their lives organized for
them by experts who knew the workers' interests better than the
workers themselves. It is particularly perverse that Cronin
should have singled out Tredegar as an example of how the
ignorant mob could not be trusted with freedom, for until it was
pushed aside in 1948, it was one of the finest primary medical
care schemes anywhere in the country.

But this is not the main point I wish to make. It is, rather, that
Cronin's pervasive paternalist view is seriously flawed. For him
the moral of the story is that people like him should be running
health and other services. His dislike of having to argue with a

committee which had irritatingly bigoted members will be shared by many. Such frustration often finds expression in the contention that 'the best committee is a committee of one'. This strikes a chord with many who have wasted their time arguing in public meetings, council meetings, parish meetings or in committees of any kind. It is a valid view in that collective judgements *are* often wrong: there is good reason to suppose that progress depends on people being free to back their own judgement against the collective view.

But this is not the argument of those who share Cronin's contempt for mutual aid. Their argument is, 'let's have only one decision being made', a view which presupposes that it can be established prior to any experience whose view will turn out to be correct. Underlying this argument is a great faith in the expert, but any such faith fails to take into account the limits of human knowledge. These limits tell us that we will be better advised to allow anyone who so wishes to back their judgement in the marketplace. For this to be possible wealth should be dispersed, so that many individuals control the resources essential to implement their ideas, whether the government of the day or powerful private agencies like it or not.

The most important result of the 1911 Act was its hidden costs – it diminished opportunities for self-organization, for self-realization, and for innovation. Both comparison with other countries and comparison between panel practice and non-panel contract practice strongly support this conclusion. We have already seen how services for women and children, who were excluded from the 1911 scheme, evolved in the market without government interference. Rooted in the false theory of political benevolence, the coercion of the 1911 scheme stunted the market in the inter-war years. But it did not succeed in completely wrecking the spontaneity of a people with a long tradition of liberty. A variety of schemes spontaneously evolved to supply medical care for all. Free care (paid for by charity) was available to those too poor to pay from their own resources; insurance of various types was available to people that wanted it; and private practice was available at a variety of fees adjusted to incomes. Some of the health schemes of the 1930s, notably the embryonic health centres – the medical institutes and medical aid societies – were admired by reformers bewitched by the potential of statism. The ironic result was that these schemes came to serve as the model for the next round of state coercion.

When the NHS was being planned in 1945 and 1946 the Friendly Societies Medical Alliance and the South Wales and Monmouthshire Alliance of Medical Aid Societies sought an assurance from the Minister of Health that they would be permitted to function under the new scheme. A meeting was arranged with Aneurin Bevan in January 1946.

Bevan began by admitting that he was 'somewhat embarrassed'. He was asked if he would like to see the alliance's statement in support of their case for continued existence. He replied: 'I know the valuable services rendered by Associations. I have been closely associated with them for many years, even from boyhood, so I cannot be told more than I already know, and it would therefore be a waste of your time and mine to go over the matter again. I will therefore outline to you the Government's Scheme.'

The ten delegates were presented with an outline of Bevan's plan. It was to be based 'primarily on health centres, a field in which the Medical Aid Societies had done valuable pioneering'. In the new health centres doctors were to be 'in consultation with each other'. Medical institute doctors 'would therefore be in isolation'. There was to be a distribution of doctors to areas in which they were most needed: 'How could we do that with your doctors?', he asked. The scheme 'left no proper place for indirect agencies' like medical institutes. But the delegates were assured that their experience would not be wasted, and told that there would be 'ample work' on the various committees concerned with administering the new scheme.

Bevan was again reminded of the comprehensive services available in Swindon and Tredegar. Were they now 'to be thrown on the scrap heap as redundant?' Bevan replied: 'I very much appreciate the splendid work you have done and are still doing. I am not emotional about Institutions but I am about people.' The Cabinet, he said, were 'determined not to have the scheme cluttered up by other agencies'. His conclusion was that: 'You have shown us the way and by your very efficiency you have brought about your own cessation' (FSMA, *Annual Report*, pp. 17–19, in PRO MH77/94).

On the eve of the NHS in June 1948 there were thirty-one

medical institutes in England. Of these, seventeen were to be taken over by existing medical officers on 5 July; in four cases the county councils were planning to take them over to run as health centres; in one case, York, the future was uncertain; and in nine cases the buildings were no longer to be used by GPs (although in one case the building was to be used as a VD clinic) (PRO MH77/94).

The four premises to be taken over by county councils to be run as health centres were the premises of the former Luton FSMI, the Great Western Railway Medic. l Fund Society of Swindon, the Gloucester FSMA, and the Gloucester Provident Dispensary (PRO MH77/95).

The health centres, which were expected to be in the forefront of NHS primary care, took a long while to materialize. It was to be many years before many health centres were built. By 1959 only ten health centres had been built since 1948. And many of the ninety-two GPs using them did not use the health centres as their main base (Parliamentary Debates, House of Commons, 1959–60, vol. 615, cols. 11–12). In May 1966, after eighteen years, only twenty-four health centres had come into existence since 1948, although an additional twenty-four had been approved and were under construction (Parliamentary Debates, House of Commons, 1966–7, vol. 728, col. 17). Since then numbers have increased rapidly.

But twenty years after the Act, there were less health centres than there had been medical institutes before 1946. Given the earlier record of expansion, it seems plausible that the market might have done a little better than the NHS.

11
The Market and the 1911 Act

Working-Class Opposition to Statism
When the 1911 Act was passed the possibility of introducing some kind of National Insurance scheme had been under discussion for well over thirty years. All such proposals had generally been resisted by the great bulk of manual workers and the organizations that represented them.

In the thirty years or so before the pensions and National Insurance legislation of 1908 and 1911, when these or similar schemes were under more or less active consideration, the possibility that the state might deny the working class the right of self-organization was openly resented. Indeed, manual workers had long argued against trusting governments to provide for the workers. One very powerful reason they advanced was that:

The great bulk of working men will always, from the very nature of the case, be excluded from an actual active part in the government of the nation, or of municipal corporations, whereas these associations [friendly societies] which have sprung from the people themselves afford numerous opportunities for those capable of governing, of exercising their capacities, and of educating themselves to fulfil such situations in the State as may from time to time be offered to them (*Foresters Miscellany*, January 1882, p. 8).

Working men, it was felt, had demonstrated that they were fit for self-government and that they needed no paternalistic state to care for them:

Working-men have now passed out of the nursery, and have been taught by personal experience the pleasures of walking upright and unaided, and are not likely to seek the assistance of the state in those matters which, from experience, they know they are capable of managing themselves.

We do not wish to be understood as throwing cold water upon any scheme intended to teach Britons the blessings of thrift, our objection is to the working-class being singled out as *the* class which requires nursing from cradle to grave; experience shows that our artisans are as capable of learning lessons from the teachings of the past as any other class, and their history of the past thirty years, as written in their own organizations, proves indisputably that they are competent, and will ultimately 'work out their own redemption' (*Foresters Miscellany*, January 1882, p. 9).

Initially voices such as these were heeded, but in 1911 as this book has shown, manual workers were singled out for paternalistic denial of liberty with its accompanying loss of prospects for self-realization and self-development. Today, few people are aware that so many manual workers were hostile to the paternalistic state. More seriously, the clear-sighted awareness of the defects of statism displayed by working-class leaders has been lost amidst the twentieth century's unquestioning faith in the benevolent potential of state power.

Before proceeding further, it will be helpful to dispense with one influential misunderstanding. For thirty years or so the late Professor Titmuss put forward an extraordinarily narrow view of a free market. For him, a free market is a situation in which there is a total absence of third-party organizations. There are only individuals. He argues that such a situation did not exist in the years before the 1911 Act. In this he is right, but to say that this means there was no free market in the sense in which the term is ordinarily applied is inexcusably misleading. The central issue in choosing between freedom and collectivism is the choice between compulsion and voluntarism. Specifically, the issue is, how much individual autonomy is to be permitted?

Titmuss' view totally ignores this distinction. For him the choice in 1911 was between kinds of collectivism: private (or bad) collectivism and public (or good) collectivism. It was a choice between 'different degrees of freedom; open or concealed power' (Titmuss, 1968, p. 238).

I will prefer to think of a free market as a situation in which effort is being made to maximize individual autonomy. The role of government is looked upon as a protective one: it seeks to maximize individual self-direction (which does not preclude joining voluntary associations) and is hedged about with safeguards against the abuse of its own power. Generally any kind of organization which can support itself can emerge.

The opposite situation (compulsory collectivism) is one in which the government monopolizes the provision of services either by direct control or by denying people the use of their own resources through taxation. To describe every kind of organization (or entity in which people combine their efforts) as collectivism, and to ignore whether or not membership of the entity is compulsory or voluntary, evades the central issue: the extent of individual autonomy.

The Accelerating Growth of Voluntary Provision Before 1911

Were the libertarian working-class leaders of the early 1900s misguided? Was their faith in the capacity of the workers to provide for themselves ill-founded? The evidence suggests not.

We have seen that between nine and nine and a half million of the twelve million persons eventually covered by the 1911 Act were already in insurance schemes. In 1910, the last full year before the 1911 Act, there were 6.6 million members of registered friendly societies, quite apart from those in unregistered societies. The rate of growth of the friendly societies over the preceding thirty years or so had been rapid and was accelerating. In 1877 registered membership had been 2.8 million. Ten years later it was 3.6 million, increasing at an average of 90,000 a year. In 1897 membership had reached 4.8 million, having increased on average by 120,000 a year. And by 1910 the figure had reached 6.6 million, having increased at an average annual rate since 1897 of 140,000 (Gosden, 1973, p. 91; Beveridge, 1948, p. 328).

Those not in registered or unregistered voluntary social insurance schemes had private charity available to them and, as a last resort, the Poor Law. Most important were the voluntary hospitals which, as we have seen, catered for one in four of the total population of London. In addition to charity there was private fee paying. This was not the preserve of the middle class, as some other writers occasionally imply. Private consultations were available at fees well within the means of most manual workers; and fee-paying was far from uncommon among working-class families. In this free market no one, therefore, went without some sort of primary medical care.

The standard of medical care has often been criticized, but the criticism is generally ill-founded, with the exception of cheap private practice. The evidence does suggest that medical practitioners who specialized as 'sixpenny doctors' do seem to have offered a clinically poor service, chiefly to the very poor.

The vast majority of manual workers could afford friendly society or other contributions, but there was a group of men in casual or otherwise irregular work who found it difficult to keep up the payments. Here was a group whose autonomy could have been enhanced by a government scheme 'o enable them to afford *insurance* instead of relying on charity.

In fact the National Insurance Act did little to help this group. Instead it coerced the majority of manual workers into a scheme which was no better, and in many respects worse, than their own spontaneous alternatives. Provision for the working poor could have been combined with a reform of the Poor Law, to enable its beneficiaries to enjoy the independence that insurance permitted in place of government charity. But the opportunity to reform the Poor Law was lost.

Provision for women and children was rising in the early years of the century. Instead of encouraging increased private insurance, or at least facilitating it, the government did nothing. Indeed, its actions were worse than nothing, the 1911 Act stifled the development of the medical institutes which were rapidly expanding family provision before 1911. And it fatally weakened the friendly societies vis-a-vis the medical profession, thus making it harder for them to continue to expand family provision against the professional resistance they were encountering in many localities.

Market Coverage: 1913–48
Chapters 9 and 10 describe the different types of primary medical care available in the curtailed market between 1913 and 1948, and consider how the earlier forms survived the 1911 Act. How many people in total were covered by charitable and insurance provision, and how many relied on fee-paying?

In Great Britain in 1939 there were 46.5 million persons. About 19 million were covered by National Insurance, leaving 25.5 million. Outpatient departments of both voluntary and public hospitals must have accounted for about 6 million, including the poor and the elderly as well as many on higher incomes; the charitable and provident dispensaries, perhaps 300,000; the lodges, 1.2 million; the medical institutes, 150,000; fee-for-service insurance, 2 million; public medical services, 1.2 million; private doctors' clubs, 100,000; and works or shop clubs, at least 3 million. On these estimates, around 14 million persons were covered by the above schemes. The remaining 11.5 million would have paid private fees out of their current incomes or their savings.

Professional Monopoly, 1913–48

Before 1911 it is very clear that doctors encountered considerable difficulty in maintaining even local monopolies. Competitive pressures were such that it was not only possible, but even somewhat attractive, for some doctors to defy the local cartel. Can the same conclusion be drawn for the period from 1913 to 1948?

Did competition have an effect on prices and conditions desired by the BMA? From 1920 the BMA policy was that contract rates should not be less than 'that which is deemed by the Council to be equivalent to that paid in respect of insured persons', although lower rates were permitted where 'special economic conditions' obtained. This policy was reaffirmed by the 1936 Representative Body. Also central to the BMA's policy was a wage limit of £250 a year, and the strategy of uniform charges and conditions within localities (mis-called 'free choice of doctor') (BMA Medico-Political Committee, Documents, 1938–9, GP107, pp. 18–19; *BMJ* Supplement, 9 January 1937, p. 22).

On prices the best available evidence is contained in the BMA surveys of 1935–6 and 1938–9. These show that many rates were below National Insurance medical benefit levels. Medical institutes, in particular, kept rates down. Low private club rates in north-east Suffolk, for instance, were said to be due to competition from the Lowestoft medical institute (BMA, Medico-Political Committee, Documents, 1936–7, MP36; General Practice Committee, 1938–9, GP107, p. 5). And the low rates of the Norwich public medical service were blamed on competition from the Norwich medical institute (BMA, Medico-Political Committee, Documents, 1936–7, MP6). The Reading public medical service had the lowest fees in the whole country and doctors there were told that this was causing the BMA's public medical services sub-committee 'considerable anxiety'. The Reading doctors told the BMA that it was impossible to raise charges because of active competition from the Amalgamated Friendly Societies of Reading.

The medical institutes only served around 140,000 non-insured persons in the late 1930s, but their influence on pay rates was much larger than these numbers suggest. Located in over sixty large towns, they offered competition throughout a large part of England. The competitive situation was such that in each town it took only one serious competitor to keep rates down, as the BMA survey shows. Because medical institutes offered such an attractive service, local BMA branches were careful not to let them achieve too much of a price advantage.

Works clubs also offered competition. In South Wales, where the medical aid societies were dominant, arrangements were said to have 'improved', (i.e. they had become less competitive) but in other areas, and notably in Yorkshire, fees were 'not satisfactory'. The branch council was demanding 4d a week for men and boys, but going rates were lower. Out of thirteen cases in the survey report, weekly rates in seven were 3d, and in three others 3½d (BMA, General Practice Committee, Documents, 1938–9, GP107, pp. 6, 9–10).

Competition from the ordinary friendly societies for children was particularly strong. In the late 1930s the friendly societies were organizing juvenile clubs 'in many areas' and were extending them to new areas. In 'many instances' the fees were said to be 'grossly inadequate' and there was an 'urgent need' to combat the activities of the friendly societies (BMA, General Practice Committee, Documents, 1938–9, GP107, p. 18). For a time a slightly lower rate of 8s 8d for juveniles had been accepted. This decision had been rescinded in 1937 and by June 1939 there had been 'considerable' improvement. But nevertheless, the BMA concluded that it was 'evident that in many areas there [was] an urgent need to combat the activities of the Friendly Societies' (ibid., p. 19). Public medical services had met with mixed results. Where it was necessary to come to an agreement with local friendly societies or trade unions, doctors found they could not unilaterally control fees. The Ashington (Northumberland) public medical service told the public medical services sub-committee in 1936 that their subscriptions could not be altered without mutual agreement between them and the local miners' union: 'We managed to get more control over it in many ways, but we are not able to alter the subscription.' Miners had, for instance, agreed to an increase to 1s 6d per fortnight during a period of prosperity, but after eighteen months fees had reverted to 1s 0d (BMA, Medico-Political Committee, Documents, 1936–7, MP6).

The policy of extending public medical services had paid off in many areas by 1939. Action to merge all contract practice had been taken 'in some areas with highly successful results'. Urging others to follow this lead the BMA survey report felt that this had: 'demonstrated that the Friendly Societies, if presented with a resolute front by the medical profession, are willing to pay adequate rates for contract practice' (ibid., p. 19). It is obvious from this that the friendly societies were still a force to be reckoned with, although the coming of National Insurance had made it easier in practice to maintain local price-fixing agreements against friendly society resistance. Even where relations were good the friendly societies kept the doctors on their toes. One doctor told the 1938 annual conference of the public medical services that an 'amicable' meeting had lately been held with friendly societies in St Albans. The leader of the friendly societies' delegation had said:

We are not fools. We know very well why you are pushing the Public Medical Service movement and why you are out to get the highest rates you can. It is because, when national health insurance is extended to dependants, you will then have something to bargain with (*BMJ Supplement*, 10 December 1938, p. 361).

And this was indeed the doctors' strategy. In 1939 the contract practice survey report said: 'While it can be pointed out that the medical profession is itself arranging and accepting contract practice at rates lower than the present NHI rates the Association would be considerably hampered in its case for even the continuance of the present NHI rates (BMA, Medico-Political Committee, 1938–9, GP107, p. 19). This shows that the state scheme encouraged upward pressure on fees in the market. Without this pressure they might have been lower.

Thus, doctors were unable to determine fees unilaterally in

the market; but had they enjoyed more success in imposing wage limits on patients and extending so-called 'free choice'? Wage limits were more widely applied, particularly as a result of the extension of public medical services. But the 1938–9 survey report was still complaining that adult friendly society members earning over £250 were admitted (ibid., p. 13). This was all the more true of the works clubs.

The BMA had pursued its policy of 'free choice' for all contract practice since the 1920 Representative Body. In June 1939 they were still complaining of their failure to achieve it. A memorandum to the public medical services sub-committee said: 'Despite the lapse of time the system of restricted choice is still operating in many, if not all, of the Divisional areas' (General Practice Committee, 1938–9, GP108).

To sum up: there were still considerable competitive pressures preventing the BMA from unilaterally fixing rates. Even against the background of government price-fixing in an important section of the market and a professional policy of seeking increases up to government rates in the private contract sector, the profession lacked the power to get its way. This applied not only to contract practice. When patients insured against medical fees the BMA was also unable to prevent doctors accepting, for instance, the two thirds contribution of the National Deposit Friendly Society in full settlement of accounts. Wage limits were not universally applied. Consumer combinations to offer countervailing power to the organized profession survived twenty years of pressure to obliterate them. Joint selection and closed panels still functioned, countermanding professional monopoly power and increasing the information flow to individual citizens.

In earlier chapters two specific theories of monopoly were tested. The evidence was found to support the second of these: the 'state capture' theory which holds that the threat of monopoly is at its height, not in a free market, but when producers have at their disposal the coercive power of the state. If the government abandons its role as protector of individual autonomy through the enforcement of impartial rules in favour of taking sides in the pursuit of specific material outcomes for identified groups, the risk of this type of monopoly becomes greater. Evidence from the 1913–48 period continues to support this conclusion.

12
Health and 'Market Failure': Some Conclusions

In the Introduction six commonly identified 'market failures' were described: externalities, lack of provision of public goods, monopoly, consumer ignorance, poverty, and the perverse incentives of insurance (moral hazard). What are the implications of the findings of this book for market failure theory?

Even the most ardent anti-marketeers do not argue that the first two of these market failures alone justify full-blooded state provision of health care. Some health care may be technically impossible to supply in a market and therefore a public good which government may finance or supply. But the examples usually given, such as the clearing of malarial swamps, are few. Negative externalities may also justify government intervention. The usual example given is that of communicable disease (Le Grand and Robinson, 1976, p. 35). The solution traditionally adopted has been free or subsidized vaccination, and in some cases compulsory vaccination. Another external cost is the danger that neither doctor nor patient may take into account the risk to third parties of communicable disease. Both doctor and patient, for example, may neglect to inform others about the risk of catching a paticular disease from the patient. Traditionally this has been resolved by compulsory notification. Intervention came early in the case of vaccination. As early as 1840 it was made available on demand free of charge through Poor Law medical officers, without pauperizing the recipient. In 1853 it was made compulsory for infants. Thus, whilst it may be possible to construct an argument for funding vaccination by compulsion, this is no argument for supplying the whole range of health care services in this manner.

Critics of the market do not generally regard external effects and its failure to supply public goods as the most serious of the market's inadequacies. Professional monopoly power is the most widely criticized problem, followed by the consumer's lack of knowledge, poverty, and the absence of normal incentives to economize due to third-party funding.

1. Monopoly and the State
One of the ironies of the present health debate is that some apologists for the NHS defend it on the ground that it offers a counterbalance to the power of the medical profession. Professor Culyer, for instance, contends that the real case for the NHS structure lies not on the demand side but on the supply side. In his view it has the potential to control the professionals who, he believes, enjoy too much power. And it can monitor their performance in the light of 'socially, not merely medically, determined objectives' (1976, p. 147). Bosanquet's view is similar. According to him, the NHS has 'above all . . . been a countervailing force to the medical monopoly'. Moreover, he contends that, 'Originally the most important part of this role was in reducing monopoly power over price' (1984, p. 49). By 'originally' he presumably means that at some historical point the NHS lowered or contained medical incomes. Bosanquet also believes that the 'NHS setting' provides a better chance of developing independent tests of clinical effectiveness run by third parties. He thinks the need for such tests is an especially strong reason for the countervailing power of the NHS (ibid., p. 50).

The available evidence suggests that generally doctors have made significant financial gains on those occasions when a major increase in government intervention has been under discussion. In 1911 and 1946 the government of the day needed professional cooperation, and paid their asking price. Subsequently doctors have found the state less easy to manipulate. In the 1920s there were confrontations between government and doctors over pay which left doctors dissatisfied, but generally, as Routh's study indicates and as the BMA's own surveys of market rates show (see above, p.181), the profession almost certainly did better than it would have done in the market (Routh, 1980, p. 60; see also Reader, 1966, pp. 192, 200; *BMJ*, 7 September 1907, p. 561; 14 September 1907, p. 648). Under the NHS the profession continued to do better than they probably would have done in the market until the late 1950s and early 1960s.

Lindsay's study shows that in the early years of the NHS doctors' pay was very attractive compared with the earnings of manual workers (1980, p. 59). Routh's comparison of the earnings of doctors, barristers, solicitors, and dentists in 1913–14, 1922–3, and 1955–6 shows that doctors' incomes increased more rapidly than those of solicitors and barristers, and by slightly less than dentists (1980, p. 60). In the early years of the NHS it may, therefore, be reasonably inferred that doctors did make significant financial gains compared with other wage and salary earners. However, the early gains made from the NHS have not been maintained and doctors' pay has tended to lag behind movements in other sectors, most notably in the early to mid 1960s and from the early 1970s onwards. It is not possible to establish satisfactorily what would have happened without the NHS, but comparison with the earnings of other groups in this country and with the incomes of medical practitioners in foreign countries suggests that doctors in Britain would probably have commanded higher incomes from the late 1950s or early 1960s onwards. There have been movements to and fro, depending on the government of the day and the extent of professional discontent. An explosion of professional feeling in the mid 1960s led to particularly large financial gains for doctors. But these proved temporary.

Monopoly power need not, of course, be used to extract only financial gains. It can be used, *inter alia*, to achieve increased leisure, to minimize accountability for medical wrongdoing, or to maximize influence on key policy decisions. There is evidence that many doctors enjoy increased leisure, and the procedure for complaining against doctors has continued to be highly unsatisfactory for the consumer. The doctors' role in decision making, both formally and in practice, has been considerable, so much so that one leading scholar describes the NHS as being under a 'syndicalist system of professional control' (Klein, 1973, p. 60). This observation has also been made by some medical practitioners. Sir Reginald Murley, a former President of the Royal College of Surgeons, for instance, has criticized the emergence of 'professional syndicalism' from the mid 1960s onwards (in Lindsay, 1980, p. iv).

Thus, the evidence suggests that from 1911 until the late 1950s the state did not act as an effective counterweight to professional power. On the contrary, in most respects it was not a counterbalance to the organized profession but the very prop on which professional dominance rested. From the evidence of the medical markets before 1911 and between 1913 and 1948, the countervailing power of the marketplace, in the form of spontaneous consumer organizations, proved more effective than the countervailing power of the state.

From the late 1950s onwards the NHS has acted as a countervailing power, successfully containing medical incomes. But this achievement has been to some extent offset by counterbalancing professional gains in the form of increased leisure, low accountability for misconduct and negligence, and a high level of influence on key political decisions. All this is quite apart from the cost to each citizen of containing health care expenditure generally below levels free individuals would probably have chosen. When the NHS has been a counterweight to professional power it has also been a counterweight to the power of the consumer, stripping individuals of the freedom to spend their own resources as they believe best.

2. Consumer Ignorance

The superiority of the doctor's knowledge is said to make consumer choice impossible. This book has shown that this claim rests on beliefs about the medical marketplace not borne out by historical investigation. Consumers in the nineteenth and early twentieth centuries did exercise choice without acting in ways which suggest that they needed to be protected from themselves. Schemes were devised to maximize the flow of information to individuals (joint selection, and approved panels); internal complaints procedures were enforced which were fair to both sides and which kept medical wrongdoing in check; costs were contained without driving standards below a reasonable level; consumers were able to influence the price of medical care, methods of delivery, and the range of services available for their flat-rate contributions. In all these respects the medical consumer's organizations for self-protection proved equally or more attractive than the paternalistic state. Indeed, the state has been the chief instrument used to limit the flow of information to consumers – by banning canvassing and advertising, and eliminating the spontaneous organizations of medical consumers.

3. The Poor

Before 1911 the poor were taken care of by the Poor Law. Ironically one of the chief factors which led to the provision of medical benefit under the 1911 Act was the criticism levelled at the existing public scheme, the Poor Law. In the event the Poor Law remained and a scheme was introduced which forced manual workers, the great majority of whom had never had recourse to the Poor Law, into a government scheme. Moreover, those that tended to be excluded from club practice (but not always, and certainly not from the medical institutes) continued to be excluded from panel practice. It was left to the marketplace to provide for them – and this was done with great success. Improved arrangements for the poor could have been made by transferring cash to them to increase their power in the marketplace. Here was a role for government. But the chance was missed.

4. Unpredictability, Insurance, and Moral Hazard

Unlike the demand for many other commodities, health care may be required unexpectedly. This means that it is advantageous to cope with health costs through insurance. But there are special difficulties about covering health costs through insurance. One weakness of risk-related health cover is that some people may be so much at risk of ill-health that no insurance organization will be able to cover them at an affordable premium. A profit-maximizing insurance company for this reason may refuse to take the old or chronically sick. Where this occurs some kind of state intervention may be justified to ensure they are not neglected. (I have suggested how this might be done in *Economic Affairs*, April 1984.)

The most important difficulty about health insurance is not this but 'moral hazard'. There are two aspects. First, once insured, the individual may have less incentive to avoid illness or accident. And second, once insured for 100 per cent cover, and more to the point, once the premiums have been paid, the individual has an incentive to 'get his money's worth'. The cost at the time of use is zero, and so the demand for health care can increase dramatically. The problem arises because the insurance agency is a third party organization. Because someone else is paying (or seems to be paying) the patient has no incentive to contain his or her demands. Sometimes the doctor too faces no incentive to contain costs. This occurs when the insurance agency agrees to pay the doctor's fees, whatever they turn out to be.

It is now acknowledged that state insurance as well as private insurance faces the problem of moral hazard. Some scholars go further and take the view that private and government insurance both suffer from moral hazard to an *equal* extent. And some draw the political conclusion that the debate about the merits of the market as against the NHS is, therefore, an irrelevance. In their view, scholars should work at improving the cost-effectiveness of the NHS instead of wasting energy arguing about the relative merits of the market and the NHS (McLachlan and Maynard, 1982, pp. 553–4).

Their conclusion that the market has little or nothing to contribute is, I suggest, not supported by the evidence. Historically criticism of medical markets has been directed, not only against 'overconsumption' (due to moral hazard) but also against 'underconsumption', due it has been argued, to competition driving doctors' fees below the level at which they could provide a clinically efficient service (see Chapter 4). McLachlan and Maynard's consideration of the NHS shows a one-sided concern with cost containment. Certainly scholars have drawn attention to 'overconsumption' due to moral hazard, but the NHS has also been heavily criticized for causing underconsumption due to a failure by governments to allocate a sufficient proportion of the proceeds of taxation to health.

I will compare, therefore, not just the methods by which the imperfect market and the imperfect NHS have coped with overconsumption resulting from moral hazard: I will ask how the imperfect market and imperfect NHS have coped with the unavoidable and endemic problem of arriving at the optimum level of health care expenditure. Which produced the least harmful side-effects, and which best permitted a prompt response to problems as they emerged?

Historically, have private and government insurance both suffered to an equal extent from moral hazard? Flat-rate cover, entitling the insured person to unlimited consultations and unlimited medicine when prescribed in return for a fixed annual fee, was widely available before 1913 and was the dominant method of National Insurance. In both cases it paid insured persons to maximize use of the service. But the financial moral hazard differed.

It differed first because doctors took a different attitude to private insurance compared with the government scheme. I have already quoted doctors comparing friendly society contract practice with National Insurance: before 1913 insured persons were poorly-paid manual workers, afterwards doctors faced, not the 'insolvent patient', but the 'solvent state insurance company' (see pp. 107–8). Pressure to raise capitation fees was the inevitable result of such a change of attitude. In the market doctors had found it difficult to raise their fees; under National Insurance it proved a much easier task.

There was another difference. The problem of costs rising rapidly due to moral hazard was encountered very early in the history of medical insurance. Nineteenth-century friendly societies had experimented with fee-for-service medical 'pools' which paid doctors' bills whenever they were presented and usually regardless of their magnitude. Many such schemes were abandoned as costs went through the roof. The solution usually adopted was to put a ceiling on the expenditure a doctor could incur. The friendly societies were third party funding agencies, but they differed from some types of insurance fund in that the doctor's budget was fixed. The societies collected, say, a penny a week from members and the doctor was paid an annual capitation fee which usually corresponded with the amount collected. He could obtain no more money from the friendly society, neither for his time nor for medicines prescribed, and so if he spent more it was at his own expense. Of course, insured persons still had no incentive to limit their demands on the doctor's time – and in practice some doctors did complain that patients called on them for 'trivial' reasons – but the cost of the doctors' fees and the cost of drugs prescribed were contained within limits working-class patients could afford.

The NHS GP service, though based on a capitation method of payment, does not enjoy the same advantages. It faces not only pressure for increased fees; the cost of medicines also has no limit and has consequently been a constant worry.

The friendly society medical institutes were formally in the same position as the NHS: they paid the drug bill, whilst the doctors were free to prescribe as they saw fit. Two factors, however, helped to contain costs in the medical institutes. Doctors were not routinely accountable for their clinical judgements (and no one in the medical institutes wanted them to be), but a doctor judged by members to be a poor performer could be rapidly dismissed. This encouraged doctors to think more carefully about the cost effectiveness of their clinical decisions. Second, the medical institutes brought doctors into a close working relationship with each institute's pharmacy staff, who naturally worked in the same building. The pharmacists tended to have more of an eye for cost than the doctors, and their physical proximity facilitated consultation over the prescribing habits of doctors whenever it seemed necessary to either. Such consultation was not uncommon in the 1930s (Waring Interview, 1984).

Some more recent schemes, offering hospital as well as GP cover, have overcome the problem of financial moral hazard. One type of organization which lacks this defect is the American health maintenance organization (HMO). HMOs are managed by doctors with a financial stake in the enterprise. Consequently they have a stronger incentive to take costs into consideration.

Ironically, the health maintenance organization is admired by Alan Maynard. Markets, he says, are seen as more efficient in allocating resources because competitive processes reward those who minimize costs and provide incentives for decision-takers to behave efficiently. But the market may be defective in the sphere of health care because professional power, the agency relationship, and the nature of insurance, tend to blunt competition, making it likely that outcomes will be 'uneconomic and not necessarily superior' to alternatives such as the NHS (Maynard, 1982, p. 488). The one institution which he feels may overcome this problem, the health maintenance organization (1982, p. 507) emerged in the (despised) American marketplace. It emerged in the market because only the market permits such innovation. Despite this Maynard believes the market–state debate is of little relevance to the problem of cost control (McLachlan and Maynard, 1982, pp. 553–4).

More orthodox insurance funds have employed a variety of devices to overcome moral hazard. Most common have been the use of co-insurance (the insurer pays only a fixed percentage of medical bills and the consumer pays the remainder) and deductibles (the consumer pays a fixed amount every time a claim is lodged or meets all his medical expenses during a quarter or year, up to an agreed maximum). However, such devices are said to impinge most on those with the least money, and this is seen by some as unjust. (This can be overcome by vouchers.) It has also been argued that co-insurance makes no difference to demand, because the doctor can increase consumption at will due to the agency relationship. But this view has been successfully criticized, and at best the evidence is inconclusive (see e.g. Newhouse, 1981).

The problem of moral hazard can afflict third-party funding agencies whether they are state or voluntary. The market has its methods of resolving the problem, as has the state. But there is a very serious risk: that of overkill. In the market there is a risk that cost-sharing devices will impinge too greatly on the poor. But this is a problem which, as I have argued, admits of relatively easy resolution. The methods by which the state has imposed limits on consumption raise far more serious problems. In this country there is little doubt that overall health care expenditure has been held below levels that people would have selected if they had enjoyed control of their own resources. As Rudolf Klein has observed, the guiding principle of the NHS is 'that health care should be provided according to need, not in response to demand'. He goes on: 'indeed, it can be argued that the real achievement of the NHS is to *minimize* the total expenditure on health care, while making rationing – which may, in some circumstances even mean turning away to die people who could be helped . . . socially and politically acceptable' (1982, p. 101).

I even go as far as to suggest that expenditure levels have been so seriously curtailed under the NHS that the number of people who have been denied health care since 1948 is almost certainly greater than it would have been if there had been no NHS. Without the safety valve of the private sector the cost of the NHS in terms of personal suffering would have been still higher than it has been. The moral point seems to be this. If there is overconsumption due to moral hazard this is not a sufficient reason for the use of the state's powers of coercion. There are devices available in the market, even if imperfect, and the side-effects of these devices are far less damaging than the side-effects of state control of overall expenditure levels. One of the side effects of state allocation of funding has been that committees now sit and put a use value on people's lives. Is Mrs Smith too old to be given a kidney transplant; or even too old to be given a dialysis machine? A use value is put on the lives of those with kidney failure, and broadly, the more useful life you have left the better your chances of being cured. For the libertarian such decisions are not the legitimate province of government. People should be free to spend their resources, or to claim on their insurance, whatever their age. Government control of funding also means that all but the very rich (or those with an employer who will pay private health insurance premiums for them) are deprived of the resources to defy government decisions to deny them health care. An elderly person, for instance, may have paid taxes and insurance contributions all his life and find that at the age of, say, sixty-two he suffers kidney failure. His payments would count for nothing, he would have no *right* to treatment. And in practice he would often not be treated. It is estimated that 2,000 people a year die unnecessarily due to kidney failure. If they had comprehensive private insurance there would be no dispute. Treatment would be automatic.

The market has also been criticized for causing underconsumption. Chapter 4 considered the argument that competition drove prices below the level at which doctors could provide an efficient service. The chief concern of that chapter was to establish exactly what the evidence was. Some wider questions about the working of the price system were left unexamined.

The chief claim made by critics of the market was that competition drove capitation fees so low that doctors were unable to provide an efficient service. The capitation fee covered both the cost of the doctor's attendance and the cost of medicines. When fees were very low it was said that doctors cut their expenditure on medicines to the detriment of patients. The evidence suggested that this occasionally happened. Can it, therefore, be concluded that underconsumption is a problem faced equally by the NHS and the market?

Compare the position of the consumer facing underconsumption in the market with the consumer facing the underconsumption of the NHS. First, what signals reached consumers in the market? In some cases doctors spoke out, openly complaining about low fees. Others refused to supply expensive drugs; and some supplied smaller quantities than they habitually supplied fee-for-service patients, thus requiring contract patients to call back if more was needed. The consumer facing these signals could adopt a number of measures: the doctor could be sacked; or he could be disciplined, perhaps fined; or the society could pay a higher fee. All these remedies were in regular use. There were occasions when doctors did not speak out, preferring to get by with a couple of cheap stock mixtures used for all but the most serious ailments. How did the consumer know he was getting a bad service in such cases? The friendly society member had available ample comparisons in the form of other society branches. The going rates were known, prevailing standards of service were known, and doctors each had a reputation for skill and attentiveness. There might also be a medical institute offering a clear alternative.

How does the position of the NHS patient compare? Doctors are free to speak out if they wish. Let us assume, therefore, equal awareness of an underconsumption problem to the extent this depends on critics speaking freely. But the knowledge of the NHS patient is impaired because comparisons are less available than they have been in past markets. More important, how effective are the remedies available to the NHS patient? The friendly society member who wanted the capitation fee raised had to persuade the branch meeting; the NHS patient has to persuade the government. Convincing, say, a hundred brothers with shared knowledge and experience of a particular doctor and of the alternatives available is a lot easier than convincing the government of the day.

Prices bargained locally between doctor and consumer offered consumers greater power to directly affect their own circumstances than the NHS ever has. Locally bargained prices were imperfect, but still preferable to the pauperization imposed by the NHS.

Any price was determined partly by how much consumers were willing and able to pay and partly by competition between suppliers. During most of the nineteenth century the ready availability of medical practitioners and consequent competition among them put consumers in most areas in a position of strength. This power was used to influence fees, but also important on the demand side was the inclination of consumers to take full advantage of their power to lower fees. I detect that in some cases at any rate, it was not considered 'the done thing' to exploit fully one's market power. Self-interest no doubt played a part in that manual workers would have known only too well that someone who felt their arm had been twisted would be unlikely to make a willing worker. But it also had to do with what consumers saw as 'fair play'.

The price, however arrived at, sent signals to potential suppliers. These might be doctors in private practice but not in contract practice; doctors working as assistants to principals and thinking of going on their own; doctors in hospitals; retired or semi-retired practitioners; young individuals contemplating a career in medicine; or medical men in contract practice looking for higher pay either in their current post or by moving elsewhere. A doctor thinking about accepting a particular post at a particular price would consider whether he could recover his outlays from the price and leave a surplus on which he could live. Each decision to supply or not to supply, in turn, had an effect on the price.

Consider the set of circumstances to which critics of the market usually draw attention: the doctor skimping on drugs because he felt the capitation fee was too low. What proportion of capitation fees was spent on drugs? When the 1911 Act came into force, 1s 6d was allocated for drugs. If this amount was spent on medicine under contract practice, what proportion was left over to cover the doctor's time? Over three quarters of friendly society capitation fees in 1905 were over 4s 0d per annum. A very common fee was 4s 4d, a penny a week. The sum 1s 6d represents just over one third of 4s 4d, a ratio of labour to materials of 2:1. Such a ratio was not unworkable. Around 15 per cent of fees were between 3s and 4s. At the lowest level, 3s 0d, this represented a fifty/fifty split between labour and materials; again, not so unworkable a ratio that it placed doctors in Titmuss' 'moral void'. In the remaining 8 per cent of cases surveyed, doctors were paid between 2s and 3s a year. For this small minority, and assuming other things to be equal, the nearer the fee was to 2s 0d the stronger the temptation to save on drugs is likely to have been. But in such cases the remedy lay in the hands of the consumer. Moreover many doctors served more than one lodge and were in a position to carry the odd low fee as long as all their fees were not that low. And many doctors were people of strong moral views who would not lightly have neglected their patients. The morality of each doctor is an independent variable in the calculation. But, let us assume the worst: that 8 per cent of friendly societies surveyed by the BMA in 1905 paid doctors' fees which made it hard for them to support their families without unreasonably cutting expenditure on drugs. Does this amount to a case for stripping the other 92 per cent of all control of their own resources?

To sum up: neither 'underconsumption' nor 'overconsumption' in the market amount to a case for the replacement of the market by the state. Overconsumption resulting from moral hazard is not a sufficient reason for using the coercive apparatus of the state. The market, with its imperfections, was better able to meet consumer wants. And the market modified by state cash transfers to the poor could ensure that everyone was covered, rich and poor alike, without exception. A state, on the experience of the NHS, which tries to provide a service direct and to finance it from taxes is less well equipped to satisfy the wants of its people.

The 'underconsumption' of the imperfect market was a lesser evil than the underconsumption of the imperfect NHS. In the market consumers retained the power to learn from experience. The NHS denies people the information to make decisions by restricting the alternatives, and more seriously, denies them the power to remedy the problems they face.

The Contemporary Relevance of the Findings

This book has found that a number of beliefs about the market are not based on the facts. One response to this might be to argue that this is fine as far as it goes, but there has been social and economic change since 1948 which makes the findings of historical interest only. Is this a valid assertion?

Certainly there has been social and economic change. For instance, there has been an advance in medical knowledge and in medical technology, but how much has this altered the essential relationship between doctor and patient? Patients have always sought the help of doctors because they were perceived as having skills or knowledge the patient wanted. This was true in 1850, and it is still true today. The content of knowledge has changed, and perhaps its complexity has also changed, but the essential character of the relationship has not. Some might say that the growth of medical knowledge has made it more difficult for the patient to possess even an inkling of the doctor's knowledge. In some limited, specialist spheres this may be true (although in such cases *most* doctors will be as ignorant as most patients). But far more importantly, it is widely recognized that a very high proportion of illnesses with which doctors now deal are the result of the way we live our lives. This notoriously applies to heart conditions and to cancer. If the individual adopts simple rules – which literally a child can understand – such as 'do not drink alcohol to excess', 'do not eat too much fat, sugar, or salt', 'take a little exercise each day', 'do not smoke cigarettes', and so on, his or her chances of remaining healthy are very substantially increased. So the growth in our understanding of what makes for good health suggests that our own private decisions about lifestyle are of central importance.

Even if this were not so, the advance in medical knowledge has not put the consumer in a weaker position vis-a-vis the doctor. Doctors have always known more than patients, and this has always made it possible for the unscrupulous practitioner to take advantage of the innocent patient. What is important is that the patient should have available ample information about the performance of particular doctors and that the patient should be powerful enough to act on this information. As this book has shown, devices to speed up the information flow to patients, to facilitate comparisons, to discipline poor performers, and to effect choices, were more widely available before the NHS than they are today.

Indeed, far from being an impediment to consumer sovereignty, modern information technology could facilitate consumer audit of primary medical care. There are even signs that elements of the medical profession are becoming more sympathetic to the education of the consumer for competition. The Royal College of General Practitioners hopes that practices will produce brochures describing their services, thus facilitating comparisons. But this infringes the GMC's advertising ban.

Changes have occurred during this century. But I suggest that these have not been so fundamental as to justify the view that the findings of this book entirely fail to help us make intelligent guesses about what the future may hold. Some of the findings may even indicate what could emerge in the future if we were more free. This is not to say that earlier institutions are likely to re-emerge exactly as they were; but some of the organizational forms that evolved spontaneously before 1948 are very likely to re-appear in suitably modern form. The election of doctors in local friendly society branch meetings, after inviting tenders, is not the strongest candidate for re-emergence. But consumer-approved panels are very likely to re-appear. We have already seen a growing interest in patient participation. The first patient participation group developed in 1971, and by January 1984 there were about fifty-five (Klein, 1984, pp. 20–21).

Specialization has been growing apace, and this is likely to continue. But this carries risks of narrow diagnosis and treatment when a more general or 'holistic' approach may be more in the patient's interests. In America GPs are a dying breed, but in this country I would expect general practice to survive as a specialism, with the family doctor emerging as a 'broker' advising patients about specialists and other options available. Legal reform would probably be necessary to ensure the strict independence of GPs from specialists and hospitals.

Changes in medical technology also facilitate the redistribution of some equipment and facilities from hospitals to health centres. Many of the services currently offered in expensive and inconvenient hospital outpatient departments will be transferred to primary health care centres.

Health maintenance organizations, with their emphasis on patient involvement and preventive medicine – screening, regular check-ups – would emerge, employing both GPs and specialists. Especially likely to occur is a great blossoming of special clinics and centres for women, whether for the 'well woman' – screening to detect breast cancer, or cancer of the cervix – or to provide for special requirements in family planning and in child birth. The power of the hospital over birth practices would decline rapidly.

The central change this century has been the monumental growth in the power of the state. This has strengthened the hand of the organized medical profession at the expense of consumers. In particular, the consumer's spontaneous organizations have been dismantled, whilst the producer's have remained. In any transition from statism to freedom, this would put the consumer at very great disadvantage, perhaps necessitating a temporary role for the government in redressing the balance. But with this qualification, what happened in previous markets of living memory could happen again. The story of working-class achievement recounted in these pages ought not to be ignored by today's public policy makers.

References

Abel-Smith, B. (1964), *The Hospitals 1800–1948*, London, Heinemann.

Abel-Smith, B. (1976), *Value for Money in Health Services*, London, Heinemann.

Ancient Order of Foresters (1915), *Formularies and Lectures*.

Armstrong, B.N. (1939), *The Health Insurance Doctor: His Role in Great Britain, Denmark and France*, Princeton, Princeton University Press.

Arrow, K.J. (1963) 'Uncertainty and the welfare economics of medical care', *American Economic Review*, vol. 53, no. 5, pp. 941–73.

BMA (1943), BMA Medical Planning Commission, *Draft Interim Report 1942*, *BMJ*, 16 January 1943.

BMA, CPR (1905), BMA Medico-Political Committee, 'An investigation into the economic conditions of contract medical practice in the United Kingdom', *BMJ Supplement*, 22 July 1905, pp. 1–96.

Beveridge, W.H. (1948), *Voluntary Action*, London, George Allen & Unwin.

Black (1980), *Inequalities in Health*, (chairman, Sir Douglas Black), London, DHSS.

Booth, C. (1902) *Life and Labour of the People in London*, First Series: Poverty (4 vols.), London, Macmillan.

Bosanquet, N. (1984) 'How to save the nation's health: the social market view', *Economic Affairs*, vol. 4, no. 3, pp. 49–50.

Brabrook, E.W. (1898), *Provident Societies and Industrial Welfare*, London, Blackie.

Brend, W.A. (1917), *Health and the State*, London, Constable.

Brown, R.G.S. (1978), *The Changing National Health Service*, 2nd edition, London, Routledge & Kegan Paul.

Bunbury, H. (1957), *Lloyd George's Ambulance Wagon*, London, Methuen.

Carr-Saunders, A.M. and Wilson, P.A. (1933), *The Professions*, London, Oxford University Press.

Cartwright, A. (1967), *Patients and Their Doctors*, London, Routledge & Kegan Paul.

Comyns Carr, A.S., Stuart Garnett, W.H., and Taylor, J.H. (1912), *National Insurance*, 1st edition, London, Macmillan.

Cooper, M. (1975), *Rationing Health Care*, London, Croom Helm.

Cox, A. (1950), *Among the Doctors*, London, Christopher Johnson, no date shown [1950].

Cronin, A.J. (1936), *The Citadel*, London, Victor Gollancz (1978 reprint).

Cullis, J.G. and West, P.A. (1979), *The Economics of Health*, Oxford, Martin Robertson.

Culyer, A.J. (1971), 'The nature of the commodity "health care" and its efficient allocation', *Oxford Economic Papers*, vol. 23, pp. 189–211.

Culyer, A.J. (1976), *Need and the National Health Service*, London, Martin Robertson.

Culyer, A.J. (1980), *The Political Economy of Social Policy*, Oxford, Martin Robertson.

Culyer, A.J. (1982) 'The NHS and the market: images and realities', in McLachlan, G. and Maynard, A., *The Public/ Private Mix For Health*, London, Nuffield Provincial Hospitals Trust, pp. 23–55.

Culyer, A.J. (1983), 'Economics without economic man', *Social Policy and Administration*, vol. 17, no. 3, pp. 188–203.

DHSS (1979), *Patients First*, London, HMSO.

DHSS (1982), *Health and Personal Social Services Statistics*, London, HMSO.

Dawson (1920), Consultative Council on Medical and Allied Services, Interim Report, *Future Provision of Medical and Allied Services*, Cmd 693. London, HMSO.

Eckstein, H. (1960), *Pressure Group Politics: the Case of the British Medical Association*, London, Allen & Unwin.

Eder, N.R. (1982), *National Health Insurance and the Medical Profession in Britain, 1913–1939*, New York and London, Garland.

Forsyth, G. (1973), *Doctors and State Medicine*, 2nd edition, London, Pitman Medical.

Friedman, D. (1978), *The Machinery of Freedom*, 2nd edition, New York, Arlington House.

GMC (1893), Report of the Committee on Medical Aid Associations, General Medical Council, *Minutes*, 1893, Appendix XII.

General Register Office (1957), Studies on Medical and Population Subjects No. 12, 'The Survey of Sickness, 1948–52', London, HMSO.

George, V. (1968), *Social Security: Beveridge and After*, London, Routledge & Kegan Paul.

Gilbert, B.B. (1966), *The Evolution of National Insurance in Great Britain*, London, Michael Joseph.

Goodman, J.C. (1980a), *National Health Care in Great Britain: Lessons for the USA*, New York, Fisher Institute.

Goodman, J.C. (1980b), 'USA: Health services are superior', in Seldon (ed) (1980), pp. 125–32.

Gosden, P.H.J.H. (1961), *The Friendly Societies in England*, Manchester, Manchester University Press.

Green, D.G. (1982), *The Welfare State: For Rich or for Poor?* IEA Occasional Paper 63, London, Institute of Economic Affairs.

Green, D.G. and Cromwell, L.G. (1984), *Mutual Aid or Welfare State. Australia's Friendly Societies*, Sydney, Allen & Unwin.

Griffiths (1983) *NHS Management Inquiry* (Chairman, E.R. Griffiths), London, DHSS.

Harris, R.W. (1946), *National Health Insurance in Great Britain 1911–1946*, London, Allen & Unwin.

Hayek, F.A. (1960), *The Constitution of Liberty*, London, Routledge & Kegan Paul.

Hayek, F.A. (1973–79), *Law, Legislation and Liberty* (3 vols.), London, Routledge & Kegan Paul.

Hodgkinson, R. (1967), *The Origins of the National Health Service: the Medical Services of the New Poor Law, 1834–71*, London, Wellcome Historical Medical Library.

ICE (1912–13) Insurance Commission (England) *Report on the Administration in England of the National Insurance Act, Part I*, London, HMSO.

ICW (1912–13) Insurance Commission (Wales), *Report on the Administration of the National Insurance Act, Part I*, London, HMSO.

IDCRGP (1946), *Report of the Inter-Departmental Committee on Remuneration of General Practitioners*, Cmd 6810, May.

Jewkes, J. and S., Kemp, A., and Lees, D.S. (1964), *Monopoly or Choice in Health Services*, IEA Occasional Paper 3, London, Institute of Economic Affairs.

Jewkes, J. and S. (1962), *The Genesis of the British National Health Service*, 2nd edition, Oxford, Blackwell.

Jones, I.M. (ed.) (1970), *Health Services Financing* (A report commissioned by the BMA; chairman, I.M. Jones), London, BMA.

Juby, B. (1980), 'Better medical attention for all in the Midlands', in Seldon (ed.) (1980), pp. 7–11.

Kessel, R.A. (1958), 'Price discrimination in medicine', *Journal of Law and Economics*, vol. 1, pp. 20–53.

Klein, Reva (1984), 'Much like an elastic stocking', *Health and Social Service Journal*, 5 January 1984, pp. 20–21.

Klein, R. (1973), *Complaints Against Doctors*, London, Charles Knight.

Klein, R. (1982), 'Private practice and public policy: regulating the frontiers', in McLachlan & Maynard (1982), pp. 95–128.

Klein, R. (1983), *The Politics of the National Health Service*, London, Longman.

Le Grand, J. (1982), *The Strategy of Equality*, London, George Allen & Unwin.

Le Grand, J. and Robinson, R. (1976), *The Economics of Social Problems*, London, Macmillan.

Lees, D.S. (1965), 'Health through choice', in Harris, R. (ed.) *Freedom or Free-for-all* (collected Hobart Papers, vol. 3), London, Institute of Economic Affairs, pp. 21–94.

Lees, D.S. (1966), *Economic Consequences of the Professions*, IEA Research Monograph 2, London, Institute of Economic Affairs.

Lees, D.S. (1976), 'Economics and non-economics of health services', *Three Banks Review*, no. 110, June, pp. 3–20.

Levitt, R. (1977), *The Reorganised National Health Service*, 2nd edition, London, Croom Helm.

Levitt, R. (1979) *The Reorganised National Health Service*, 2nd edition, revised, London, Croom Helm.

Levy, H. (1943), 'The economic history of sickness and medical benefit before the Puritan Revolution', *Economic History Review*, vol. 13, pp. 42–57.

Levy, H. (1944a), 'The economic history of sickness and medical benefit after the Puritan Revolution', *Economic History Review*, vol. 14, pp. 135–60.

Levy, H. (1944b), *National Health Insurance: A Critical Study*, Cambridge, Cambridge University Press.

Lindsay, C.M. et al. (1980), *National Health Issues: the British Experience*, London, Hoffman La Roche.

Lindsay, C.M. (ed.) (1980), *New Directions in Public Health Care*, 3rd edition, San Francisco, Institute for Contemporary Studies.

Lindsay, C.M. and Buchanan, J.M. (1970), 'The organization and financing of medical care in the United States', in Jones (1970), pp. 535–85.

Little, E.M. (1932), *History of the British Medical Association 1832–1932*, London, BMA.

MOH (1919–20), *Annual Report of the Chief Medical Officer*, Cmd 978, London, HMSO, 1920.

Maynard, A. (1982), 'The regulation of public and private health care markets', in McLachlan, G. and Maynard, A. (eds) (1982), pp. 471–512.

Maynard, A. and Ludbrook, A. (1980), 'What's wrong with the National Health Service?', *Lloyds Bank Review*, October, pp. 27–41.

Maynard, A. and Ludbrook, A. (1981), 'Thirty years of fruitless endeavour? An analysis of government intervention in the health care market', in Van der Gaag and Perlman (eds) (1981), pp. 45–65.

McConaghey, R.M.S. (1966), 'Medical practice in the days of Mackenzie', (The James Mackenzie Memorial Lecture) *The Practitioner*, vol. 196, pp. 147–60.

McLachlan, G. and Maynard, A. (eds) (1982), *The Public/Private Mix For Health*, London, Nuffield Provincial Hospitals Trust.

Mechanic, D. (1968), 'General Practice in England and Wales', *Medical Care*, vol. 6, no. 3, May–June, pp. 245–60.

Merrison (1975), *Report of the Committee of Inquiry into the Regulation of the Medical Profession*, Cmnd 6018, London, HMSO.

Mill, J.S. (1970), *Principles of Political Economy*, Harmondsworth, Penguin.

Mill, J.S. (1972), *Utilitarianism, On Liberty, and Considerations on Representative Government*, London, Dent.

Monopolies Commission (1970), *A report on the general effect on the public interest of certain restrictive practices so far as they prevail in relation to the supply of professional services*, Cmmd 4463, London, HMSO.

NHIJC (1917), National Health Insurance Joint Committee, *Report on the Administration of National Health Insurance 1914–17*, London, HMSO.

Newhouse, J.P. (1978), *The Economics of Medical Care: A Policy Perspective*, Reading, Mass., Addison-Wesley.

Newhouse, J.P. (1981), 'The demand for medical care services: a retrospect and a prospect', in Van der Gaag, J. and Perlman, M. (eds), *Health, Economics, and Health Economics*, Amsterdam, North-Holland.

Nozick, R. (1974), *Anarchy, State, and Utopia*, London, Blackwell.

Orr, D.W. and J.W. (1938), *Health Insurance with Medical Care: The British Experience*, New York, Macmillan.

PEP (1937), *Report on the British Health Services*, London, Political and Economic Planning.

PMSUP (1910), *Report as to the Practice of Medicine and Surgery by Unqualified Persons in the United Kingdom*, Cd 5422, London, HMSO.

Paine, T. (1976), *Common Sense*, Harmondsworth, Penguin.

Pater, J.E. (1981), *The Making of the National Health Service*, London, King Edward's Hospital Fund for London.

Peterson, M.J. (1978), *The Medical Profession in Mid-Victorian London*, Berkeley, University of California Press.

Plender (1912), *Report of Sir William Plender to the Chancellor of the Exchequer on the result of his investigation into existing conditions in respect of medical attendance and remuneration in certain towns*. Cd 6305, London, HMSO.

Pride, S. (1923), *Glimpses of History* (Private pamphlet published to celebrate the 80th anniversary of court Benevolence 1594, AOF.) Luton, AOF.

RCAP (1895), *Royal Commission on the Aged Poor*, C. 7684, London, HMSO.

RCFS (1874), *Royal Commission on Friendly and Benefit Building Societies*, London, HMSO.

RCL (1893), *Royal Commission on Labour*, London, HMSO.

RCNHI (1926), *Royal Commission on National Health Insurance*, London, HMSO.

RCNHS (1979), *Royal Commission on the National Health Service*, Cmnd. 7615, London, HMSO.

RCPL (1909), Royal Commission on the Poor Laws and Relief of Distress, *Report*, London, HMSO.

RCPL, MR (1909), Royal Commission on the Poor Laws and Relief of Distress, *Minority Report*, London, HMSO.

Reader, W.J. (1966), *Professional Men*, London, Weidenfeld & Nicolson.

Ritchie, D.G. (1891), *The Principles of State Interference*, London, Swan Sonnenschein.

Ross, J.S. (1952), *The National Health Service in Great Britain*, London, Oxford University Press.

Rothbard, M. (1978), *For a New Liberty: the Libertarian Manifesto*, 2nd edition, New York, Collier.

Rothschild (1898), *Report of the Committee on Old Age Pensions*.

Routh, G. (1980), *Occupation and Pay in Great Britain 1906–79*, 2nd edition, London, Macmillan.

Rowntree, B. Seebohm (1901), *Poverty: A Study of Town Life*, London, Macmillan.

Rumsey, H.W. (1856), *Essays on State Medicine*, London, John Churchill.

SCADP (1899), Select Committee on the Aged Deserving Poor, *Report and Minutes of Evidence*, July.

SCMPR (1844), *Select Committee on Medical Poor Relief*, London, HMSO.

Schumpeter, J. (1976), *Capitalism, Socialism and Democracy*, 5th edition, London, George Allen & Unwin.

Scotton, R.B. (1974), *Medical Care in Australia: an Economic Diagnosis*, Melbourne, Sun.

Seldon, A. (1977), *Charge*, London, Temple Smith.

Seldon, A. (ed) (1980), *The Litmus Papers: A National Health Dis-service*, London, Centre for Policy Studies.

Seldon, A. (1968), *After the NHS* (Occasional Paper 21), London, IEA.

Siddall, T.W. (1924), *Story of a Century*, Sheffield, 100F, MU, Sheffield District.

Smith, A. (1776), *The Wealth of Nations*, Everyman edition (1977), London, Dent.

Smith, H.L. (1819), *Observations on the Prevailing Practice of Supplying Medical Assistance to the Poor, Commonly called the Farming of Parishes with Suggestions for the Establishment of Parochial Medicine Chests or Infirmaries in Agricultural Districts*, London (British Library: 1028.i.3(1).)

Smith, H.L. (1825), *The Second Annual Report of the Southam Dispensary* (British Library: 1028.i.3(2).)

Smith, H.L. (1830), *Abstract of a Plan for the Formation of Self-Supporting Charitable and Parochial Dispensaries*, c.1830 (British Library: 1488.cc.11.)

Stevens, R. (1966), *Medical Practice in Modern England*, New Haven and London, Yale University Press.

Stimson, G. and Webb, B. (1975), *Going to see the Doctor*, London, Routledge & Kegan Paul.

Stewart, W.H. and Enterline, P.E. (1961), 'Effects of the National Health Service on physician utilization and health in England and Wales', *New England Journal of Medicine*, vol. 265, no. 24, pp. 1187–94.

Sugden, R. (1983), *Who Cares?* IEA Occasional Paper 67, London, IEA.

Styrap, J. de (1895), *A Code of Medical Ethics*, 4th edition, London, H.K. Lewis.

Thomas, K.B. (1974), 'Temporarily dependent patient in general practice', *British Medical Journal*, 30 March, pp. 625–6.

Titmuss, R.M. (1959), 'Health' in Ginsberg, M. (ed.), *Law and Opinion in England in the 20th Century*, London, Stevens & Sons, pp. 299–318.

Titmuss, R.M. (1963), *Essays on the Welfare State*, 2nd edition, London, Allen & Unwin.

Titmuss, R.M. (1968), *Commitment to Welfare*, London, Allen & Unwin.

Turner, E.S. (1958), *Call the Doctor*, London, Michael Joseph.

Waring (1984), Interview with C.J. Waring, Secretary of the Norwich Friendly Societies Medical Institute 1939–48, and previously Assistant Secretary.

Webb, B. (1975), *Our Partnership*, Cambridge, Cambridge University Press.

Webb, S. and B. (1910), *The State and the Doctor*, London, Longman.

Williams, A. (1978), 'Need – an economic exegesis', in Culyer, A.J. and Wright, K.G. (eds), *Economic Aspects of Health Services*, London, Martin Robertson, pp. 32–45.

Wood, G.H. (1962), 'Real wages and the standard of comfort since 1850', in Carus-Wilson, E.M. (ed.), *Essays in Economic History*, London, Edward Arnold.

Wood, P. (1980), 'Better medical attention for all: in Southern England', in Seldon (ed.) (1980), pp. 13–20.

Periodicals

Ancient Order of Foresters, Quarterly Reports
Association Medical Journal
British Medical Journal
Foresters Directory
Foresters Miscellany
Lancet
Monthly Review of Friendly Societies
National Insurance Gazette
Oddfellows Magazine

Index